This is a beautifully written, accessible book that... parenting—"balanced parenting"—that will... help par... raising their kids, even in the face of adversity. And, unlike many fads and fashions in parenting that come and go with the times, these authors' recommendations are grounded in decades of solid, scientific research. I love this book!

–LAURENCE STEINBERG, PhD, DISTINGUISHED UNIVERSITY PROFESSOR OF
PSYCHOLOGY AND NEUROSCIENCE AT TEMPLE UNIVERSITY,
PHILADELPHIA, PA; AUTHOR OF *YOU AND YOUR ADULT CHILD:
HOW TO GROW TOGETHER IN CHALLENGING TIMES*

An excellent addition to our understanding of the role that both adverse and protective childhood experiences play in the development of resilience. I highly recommend this balanced approach to parenting to anyone raising children, and especially those who either had adverse experiences in their own childhood or who are parenting children who had them.

–MICHAEL H. POPKIN, PhD, COUNSELING PSYCHOLOGY; FOUNDER AND
PRESIDENT, ACTIVE PARENTING PUBLISHERS; AUTHOR OF *THE ACTIVE
PARENTING PROGRAMS*

Amanda Sheffield Morris and Jennifer Hays-Grudo provide parents with a compelling and engrossing introduction to the scientific research on parenting. They explain how balanced parenting, which involves age-appropriate levels of warm support and limit-setting, best promotes resilience and illustrate this approach concretely in relation to children of different ages, including those who have experienced adversity. Morris and Hays-Grudo are both developmental psychologists as well as parents who use their varied experiences and expertise to maximal effect.

–MICHAEL E. LAMB, EMERITUS PROFESSOR OF PSYCHOLOGY AND FELLOW,
SIDNEY SUSSEX COLLEGE, UNIVERSITY OF CAMBRIDGE, CAMBRIDGE,
ENGLAND; EDITOR OF *PSYCHOLOGY, PUBLIC POLICY, & LAW*

Raising a Resilient Child

in a World of Adversity

in a World of Adversity

Raising a Resilient Child

in a World of Adversity

Effective Parenting for
Every Family

Amanda Sheffield Morris PhD
& Jennifer Hays-Grudo PhD

 AMERICAN PSYCHOLOGICAL ASSOCIATION

The opinions and statements published are the responsibility of the authors, and such opinions and statements do not necessarily represent the policies of the American Psychological Association.

Published by
APA LifeTools
750 First Street, NE
Washington, DC 20002
https://www.apa.org

Order Department
https://www.apa.org/pubs/books
order@apa.org

Typeset in Sabon by Circle Graphics, Inc., Reisterstown, MD

Printer: Sheridan Books, Chelsea, MI
Cover Designer: Mark Karis

Library of Congress Cataloging-in-Publication Data

Names: Morris, Amanda Sheffield, author. | Hays-Grudo, Jennifer, author.
Title: Raising a resilient child in a world of adversity : effective
    parenting for every family / Amanda Sheffield Morris, PhD and
    Jennifer Hays-Grudo, PhD.
Description: Washington, DC : American Psychological Association, [2024] |
    Includes bibliographical references and index.
Identifiers: LCCN 2023020373 (print) | LCCN 2023020374 (ebook) |
    ISBN 9781433834073 (paperback) | ISBN 9781433834080 (ebook)
Subjects: LCSH: Parenting. | Resilience (Personality trait) in children.
Classification: LCC HQ755.8 .M649 2024 (print) | LCC HQ755.8 (ebook) |
    DDC 649/.1--dc23/eng/20230501
LC record available at https://lccn.loc.gov/2023020373
LC ebook record available at https://lccn.loc.gov/2023020374

https://doi.org/10.1037/0000385-000

Printed in the United States of America

10 9 8 7 6 5 4 3 2 1

We dedicate this book to our children, who taught us more about parenting than anyone else: Zack, Amy, Caleb, and Mollie.

CONTENTS

Contents

ACKNOWLEDGMENTS

Our husbands, Michael Morris and Doron Grudo, provided unflagging and enthusiastic support as we wrote this book. We could not have written this book without them or parented our children as well without them as partners. We thank our children for giving us permission to share some of our family stories. We love that Zack wrote his own version of a story for Chapter 7 (an important perspective!), and Amy shared her wisdom on parenting LGBTQ youth that we present in Chapter 6. We are grateful to our PACEs research lab for helping us shape and refine our ideas and who edited versions of this book: Jens Jespersen, Devin Barlaan, Lana Beasley, Erin Ratliff, and Jenny Watrous. We appreciate Amy Williamson, our colleague and friend, for sharing her parenting advice on a topic that can be challenging for many. Joli Jensen, author of *Write No Matter What*, appeared in our lives at the perfect time with friendship and practical advice for how to keep moving when the writing got tough. We thank our friends at https://WholeHearted.org, A. J. Foxx, Tom White, and Lukas Foxx, for helping us find our voice and reach a broader audience. Sincere thanks also to Chris Kelaher and Judy Barnes at the American Psychological Association for their support throughout the process. We acknowledge that this book is based on decades of developmental research that informed our thinking and ideas on parenting. We stand on the shoulders of those who came before us. We thank Ann Masten for giving us the courage to develop the PACEs framework, Suniya Luthar for encouraging us to be brave, and Hiram Fitzgerald for pushing us to think about the bigger and broader world in which we live.

Raising a Resilient Child

in a World of Adversity

INTRODUCTION

The hardest and most important job that any of us will ever have is being a parent. It is especially challenging when your own childhood was less than ideal. More than half of parents today experienced physical or emotional abuse, neglect, divorce, family violence, alcohol or drug abuse, or mental illness in their homes when they were children or adolescents. In the last 20 years, scientists have learned that these adverse childhood experiences, or ACEs, have lifelong consequences on physical health, mental health, and parenting. No parent wants to continue this pattern of adversity, but it is often difficult to know how to break the cycle. In this book, you will learn five essential steps to breaking the intergenerational cycle of adversity. Breaking this cycle is not easy. It involves reflecting on your past and making changes in yourself and how you parent. This book is your guide as you chart a new course, creating a home that supports your child's growth and well-being along with your own.

We all want our children to have a happy childhood. We also want them to have a childhood that prepares them to thrive in a world of adversity. In other words, we want them to be resilient. Raising resilient children is a matter of balance: giving them freedom to explore while keeping them safe, allowing them independence while staying connected, and letting them make mistakes while helping them succeed. We call this *balanced parenting*. It focuses on the parent–child relationship, keeping in mind the competing demands of children's development and parents' need for control. Certainly, there are many situations in which parents should be in control. But just as important, children need opportunities to learn and grow and become independent.

This book provides strategies for managing these balancing acts. You will learn effective ways to discipline your child, communicate better with your adolescent, and establish routines and habits in your family that naturally build children's character and resilience. Along the way, you will also become more resilient, be better able to handle your emotions and control your reactions to difficult situations, and create the life you want for you and your family.

This book is for all parents, especially those who have experienced childhood adversity or whose children have a history of trauma. We use the term *parents* throughout the book, but we acknowledge that all families are different. Parents can be mothers, fathers, stepparents, or grandparents, and many other people play important roles in children's lives. We believe you will benefit from the knowledge and experiences we share in this book at any stage of parenting—whether during pregnancy, infancy, early childhood, the teenage years, or when becoming a grandparent. We encourage you to read all the chapters, no matter your age or the age of your child. There are helpful tools and strategies for managing stress and adversity throughout the book, and you will benefit from thinking about how to promote resilience and healing at all ages and stages across the life span.

Some psychologists believe you cannot be resilient unless you have experienced trauma or significant hardship. How can you show evidence of resilience if you have never experienced adversity? While there is logic in this argument, we believe that individuals can build the capacity for resilience whenever adversity occurs. All of us will experience adversity at some point in our lives because life is hard.

If it isn't today, chances are it will be tomorrow. In this book, we focus on ways to help our children and ourselves build the potential for resilience so we are prepared when adversity comes.

We are developmental psychologists who have studied parenting, adversity, resilience, and child development for multiple decades. We have also learned many lessons from raising our own children. We have drawn on our experiences and scholarly knowledge in writing this book. We share many of the challenges we had as parents, with the permission and blessings of our children.

We recognize as developmental psychologists that parenting should differ for children at different ages. While many of the principles of good parenting are the same across ages, the emphases and strategies that work best need to change as children grow and develop. You will see in this book that we have separate chapters for parenting children at different stages of development. We begin every chapter with a story. We include practical tips, zooming-in boxes that give a little more detail on the research on child development, and recaps and activities to help you digest and use the information presented in this book. We also include Parenting Strategies for Building Resilience, proven strategies that help you and your child get from one stage to the next. Each chapter includes information on how parents' and children's exposures to trauma can lead to parenting and developmental challenges and how to create age-appropriate protective experiences to counter those effects. We provide activities to bring the parenting strategies and trauma recovery lessons to life. One of the most important things we have learned in our research is that pretending that hardship, trauma, or adverse experiences never happened is the least effective path to recovery—for adults as well as for children. Traumatic experiences do not need to be relived to be acknowledged, but they must be acknowledged to be healed.

We recognize that this book is based on our knowledge, experience, and understanding of parenting. Many families experience the intersection of racism, discrimination, poverty, illness, adversity, and other significant hardships. We acknowledge that the perspectives we share in this book are limited and biased despite our best efforts. We share many perspectives but also have our own views and have had different life experiences. Our goal is to blend and harmonize these perspectives into a coherent set of guidelines with examples from our experiences as parents and researchers. This book is the result of our desire to share what we have learned.

We live in a world of adversity. Today, parents face new challenges, such as protecting children from harmful online content, limiting their screen time, dealing with the availability of lethal and highly addictive drugs, and increasing pressures to succeed in school despite limited options for many young adults. It is not yet known what the full extent of the COVID-19 pandemic will be on this generation of children and adolescents. To be sure, we expect there will be some enduring effects, much like there were for the children of the Great Depression who were raised in the 1930s. We truly hope that some of the long-term effects of the pandemic will be positive and protective in times of future adversities. We must remember that the children who grew up during the Great Depression became known as the "Greatest Generation" for their resilience and grit. It is our hope that by reading this book, parents and future generations will benefit from understanding the many different pathways to promote resilience in themselves and their children despite what is going on in the world.

We use the analogy of a road trip throughout this book. Parenting is an epic journey with many twists and turns, detours, roadblocks, and obstacles along the way. So, get ready for this amazing trip. Pack your bags, get your map and compass, buckle your seat belt, and set out for this great adventure. It is sure to be a memorable ride—full of adventure, discovery, and resilience.

CHAPTER I

BALANCED PARENTING: THE SECRET TO RAISING A RESILIENT CHILD

Sitting on the floor late one Friday night, surrounded by baby toys and baskets of laundry, Emma realized that she had lost all control of her life when the twins were born. Almost overnight she had become responsible for the survival of two tiny humans who could do nothing to ensure their survival except coo and cry. True, they were adorable, and the intensity of her love for them often surprised her, but the demands were unrelenting. Deep down, she knew that she and her partner didn't really know what they were doing. They were just making this parenting business up as they went along, and she feared they would get it all wrong. Even if they could figure this parenting thing out, would she ever have time to watch a movie again or take a long bath? How was it possible to keep her sanity while somehow making sure these precious but helpless little creatures became competent and happy adults?

Across town, Roosevelt sat at the empty kitchen table watching the clock and worrying whether he should have let his 17-year-old son drive himself and his younger sister to the high school football game. Now they are 30 minutes late getting home, and the news is full of accidents on the freeway. Sure, his son is a good driver and has always been responsible and protective of his sister, but since Roosevelt and his wife divorced a year ago, his son is often moody and doesn't want to communicate. Worse, he has stopped having his long-time friends over for pizza and games. He just shrugs and mumbles when asked about them. His grades have suffered during the last year as well. How can he keep tabs on this almost-grown son without treating him "like a baby" and driving him further away? How can he possibly grant him the independence he craves without opening the door to all the possible missteps and mistakes that could have lifelong consequences, especially when the boy won't talk with him?

Everyone who has been a parent knows these late-night worries, the thoughts and fears that feed on our doubts about our ability to handle the physical and mental demands of raising children. As we rock colicky newborns, sit in steamy bathrooms with croupy babies, or try to lower the dangerously high temperature of a feverish toddler, we worry that we might not be up to the task. Just keeping these small explorers safe from the everyday dangers of electrical outlets, sharp objects, and stairs can feel overwhelming. As they grow older, we try to prevent the bumps and bruises of learning to walk and run, help them learn how to resolve conflicts with their siblings and friends, look both ways when they cross a street, and do well when they enter school. As they become teenagers, the days and evenings are even busier, filled with homework, arguments over screen time, and after-school activities. Parenting shifts into staying close while letting go, monitoring who they're spending time with while allowing them more independence and opportunities to explore the larger world.

When parents have experienced adversity or trauma during childhood, parenting can become even more challenging. Scientists have identified 10 types of trauma that occur between birth and age 18, called ACEs, or adverse childhood experiences. These include physical, sexual, or emotional abuse; physical or emotional neglect; divorce; domestic violence; or parental alcohol or substance abuse, criminality, or mental illness. In thousands of studies around the world, ACEs have been found to increase the risk of cancer, heart disease, depression, drug or alcohol use, and other physical and mental health problems (see Chapter 2 for more on ACEs). ACEs can also affect parenting. Having a history of ACEs may decrease your ability to manage your stress and emotions, which can limit your success in helping children manage theirs. Growing up with ACEs can also limit our understanding of how to create a healthy, nurturing home, the home we wished we'd had as children and teens. This book provides specific examples of how to overcome the effects of ACEs on parenting and offers guidelines and suggestions on how to recover from your own childhood adversities while raising resilient children.

When children have ACEs, their behavior is likely to be more challenging and require even more skill and patience from their parents. Children who have experienced abuse, neglect, divorce, domestic violence, parent mental illness, addiction, or incarceration often need additional support and guidance to overcome the biological and behavioral responses to stress caused by ACEs. The goal of every parent whose child has experienced adversity is to help them develop resilience and minimize the negative effects of those experiences. Most of the parenting strategies that promote resilience are the same strategies that have been found to help all children develop to their fullest potential. Sometimes, however, parents need additional support or resources to provide nurturance during emotionally difficult situations and ways to better respond to their children's challenging behaviors. In later chapters, we provide resources for situations that require additional professional support and assistance and suggest ways to connect with other parents seeking to break the cycle of adversity, helping their children and themselves become strong and resilient.

Our job as parents is to help our children grow up to be healthy, happy, and successful adults, however we define that. We often lose sight of this long-term goal while dealing with the constant challenges of daily life. When children are little, there never seems to be enough time to sit back and ask yourself what you want most for this child to have or be as an adult. What qualities can you help them develop that will lead to a lifetime of health and happiness? If they've experienced trauma, how do you help this child heal? How can you be the parent you didn't have? As scientists and parents, we are convinced that the surest way to help our children live happy and healthy lives is to help them develop the qualities, habits, and skills that promote resilience. Why resilience? Being resilient means being able to handle the difficulties, setbacks, and hardships that all of us will encounter at some time in our lives. Some children come into families with a long history of adversity, inheriting intergenerational patterns of pain and dysfunction. Despite their parents' best intentions, they may experience trauma and stress early in their lives. Others may not encounter adversity or hardship until they are grown. But everyone benefits from being resilient and able to cope with challenges whenever they occur. Resilience is not something we are born with but something we develop, like a muscle that gets stronger with use. When we help our children develop the attitudes, routines, habits, and skills that promote resilience, we prepare them to navigate life's hazards whenever they occur.

PARENTS AS THE HEROES OF AN EPIC JOURNEY

Preparing children to deal with potential hardship and unexpected adversity is a theme stretching back to the beginnings of time. Throughout human history and around the world, parents have passed stories from one generation to the next about heroes and heroines who face and overcome the dangers posed by mythical beasts, ruthless villains, and wicked stepmothers. In myths, fairy tales, and even today's comics, cultures have created a rich legacy of stories and visual images to prepare children for the perilous road ahead.

By telling (and retelling) the stories of Little Red Riding Hood and the Three Little Pigs at bedtime to our children, we acknowledge the dangers lurking in the forest and ways to overcome them by finding the hunter to scare off the wolf or by building a house of bricks that will withstand the wolf's attacks. The stories published in modern children's books are pale replicas of the horrors of their original versions published by the Brothers Grimm because life is (thankfully) less hazardous for most children today than it was centuries ago. But the stories persist in popularity because they communicate an essential truth known to all parents and children: Life is often dangerous, and being able to meet danger with strength, courage, and confidence is the key to a happy, healthy life.

In these classic and time-tested stories, sometimes the heroes return safely home, and sometimes the destination is a new and better home, but the destination is always a place where one is safe and loved. Reaching this destination is everyone's goal, but when we become parents, we embark on a new journey with a new goal—preparing and helping our children reach that destination. Often, it seems that we have not yet reached our destination—complete with a brick house safe from the big, bad wolf—before we are responsible for helping the next generation gain the skills and courage to build their own brick houses. In fact, becoming a parent is likely to remind us of how far we have to go to reach that sense of safety and security. Caring for our children can trigger memories and feelings from childhood that remind us just how unsafe we felt as children and how easily those painful childhood memories and feelings can be revived. For this reason, having and caring for children helps many parents recover from their traumatic childhoods and gain the skills and habits that promote resilience.

Parents who experienced abuse or neglect as children are typically highly motivated to do whatever it takes so that their own children do not repeat those experiences but instead feel safe, secure, and loved. This often requires learning parenting and relationship skills that parents did not experience or observe growing up, but these skills can be learned! In fact, most parents—with or without a history of adversity—spend a good deal of time searching for ways to deal with children's behavioral and developmental needs. We all recognize that when we can minimize conflict and increase cooperation and caring among family members, our everyday lives are happier. In later chapters, we describe steps that parents can take to help their children grow up to be resilient, regardless of what their own childhoods were like and in spite of what trauma their children may already have had. In this chapter, we focus on preparing ourselves for this parenting journey.

BALANCED PARENTING: THE KEY TO RESILIENCE

Balanced parenting is how we describe staying on course as we travel this heroic journey of parenting children along the road to resilience. *Balanced parenting* is defined as managing the competing demands of children's development with parents' need for control. This balancing act looks different at different ages but is consistent and steady overall, providing stable boundaries that allow children to explore within limits, freedom to choose within reason, and opportunities to learn on their own but with help when needed. Balanced parenting builds on and extends previous theories of parenting to guide parents who are raising children after adversity—their own or their children's.

One parenting approach that influenced us personally and professionally was Dr. Diana Baumrind's research on the link between parenting styles and children's behavior. Beginning in the 1960s, she observed that the behavior of preschool children was predicted by their parents' behavior. For example, she noted that the preschool children who were curious, happy, and well-liked by their peers and teachers had parents who treated them differently than preschoolers who were fearful and withdrawn or those who were impulsive and often in trouble. She described the parents of the well-adjusted children as *authoritative* because they managed to be both warm and communicative while also setting high expectations and predictable consequences for misbehavior. The parents of withdrawn and fearful children, whom she described as *authoritarian,* set consequences and had high expectations for their children but were not as nurturing or communicative. The parents of the children who lacked self-control were just the opposite of the authoritarian parents. They were warm and communicative but were lax in setting rules and consequences (Baumrind, 1971).

After studying parenting and particularly the benefits of *authoritative* parenting for many years, we think an additional concept is needed to help parents find that "sweet spot" where children feel safe and supported but also know that there are clear boundaries, rules, and consequences. Balanced parenting helps both parents and children recover from adversity. It emphasizes different balancing acts needed for children of different ages. It also adds the concept of balancing caring for children with parents' need to care for themselves. When parents do not balance self-care with childcare, they may find themselves losing patience, saying or doing things they later regret, and generally resorting to less effective parenting strategies. Like the flight attendant's advice to passengers to put on their own oxygen masks before helping the children flying with them, parents need to prioritize themselves as well as their children as they create family routines, expectations, and habits.

Balanced parenting involves avoiding extremes in our thinking and our behavior with children. For example, toddlers need freedom to explore, but they also need to be kept safe from harm as they learn about their world. Newborns need continuous and responsive care, but mothers and other primary caregivers also need to sleep, eat, and shower. Parenting consists of a series of balancing acts that change over time—balancing the baby's and young child's needs with the needs of parents and other family members and balancing the older child's and teen's need to spend more time with peers while staying connected to the family. This is an essential aspect of learning to live in harmony with others—other family members, friends, and society. Another aspect of parenting involves balancing children's need for autonomy and exploration with the equally important need to be protected from the harmful consequences of their actions, the actions of others, and the dangers inherent in the world. The concept of balanced parenting helps us reconcile the push–pull dynamic of wanting to hold our children close while knowing we also need to let them go. It reminds us that we are responsible as parents for encouraging them to learn and develop skills we know they will need in life while at the same time giving them opportunities to choose the goals that they want to pursue.

Balanced parenting is especially important when children have experienced trauma or significant adversity. Parenting can be challenging even in the most ideal circumstances, but parenting children who struggle to control their emotions and behavior because of trauma can be even more difficult. All children, but especially those who have experienced trauma and adversity, need to feel safe as well as be kept safe from further harm. At the same time, they also need to have opportunities to explore and engage with their physical and social environments. If preventing harm is a parent's only consideration, they limit the child's opportunity to learn, make friends, and develop a sense of competence. Likewise, when a parent is so focused on immediately meeting a child's every want or need, it prevents the child from learning how to wait or delay gratification, and it negatively affects the parent's ability to meet their own needs or the needs of others in the family. In Chapter 2, we share strategies for creating environments that promote resilience and recovery from trauma. We call these protective and compensatory experiences (PACEs) and provide specific strategies for promoting PACEs at different ages in subsequent chapters.

One of Jennifer's favorite parenting stories comes from her brother, who was driving his young family to Thanksgiving late one night on a lonely country road with narrow shoulders that dropped steeply on each side into a Louisiana swamp. Looking around and seeing that his wife and four young children were all asleep, he had a moment of panic when he realized what would happen if he, too, fell asleep and veered too far to the right or left. He found himself wondering, "Why am I driving? Why isn't Dad driving?" only to realize that now he WAS Dad! Most parents will have one of these moments when they realize they are now the generation in charge, responsible for ensuring that their families safely reach their destinations, even when it involves driving on narrow roads late at night with alligators lurking in the swamp below the road. Balanced parenting provides guidelines for staying on the road, avoiding the hazards of veering too far to one extreme or the other, avoiding being too lenient or too strict, too worried or too unconcerned, too involved or not involved enough. In Table 1.1, we describe the principles of balanced parenting, contrasting them with more extreme forms of harsh and indulgent parenting. We use these principles in later chapters to illustrate balanced parenting for children at different ages.

BALANCED PARENTING AND CHILD DEVELOPMENT

Throughout life, all of us must navigate specific social and emotional challenges that set the stage for our future development and well-being. Successfully resolving one set of challenges prepares us to meet the next set (see Erikson, 1993). Parents can help children successfully navigate these challenges by finding the right balance

TABLE 1.1. Principles of Balanced Parenting Across Ages

Harsh or anxious parenting	Balanced parenting	Indulgent or disengaged parenting
Focuses on extreme punishment	Establishes logical consequences for misbehavior	Has little or no consequences
Is overly watchful (hovering, intrusive)	Is appropriately involved in child's life	Grants independence without monitoring
Severely limits exploration	Allows exploration within limits	Sets few limits on exploration
Is self-focused and not responsive to child	Is responsive to the child while maintaining care for self and others	Indulges child's needs at the expense of caring for self
Withholds affection or makes it contingent on behavior	Delights in the child but enforces rules and consequences	Avoids criticism and feedback

between doing too much and too little, being too involved and not involved enough. As children resolve each of these developmental tasks, they acquire the internal beliefs and attitudes that form the building blocks of resilience. Table 1.2 shows the relationship between balanced parenting and resilient outcomes at each stage of development in childhood and adolescence. We briefly describe balanced parenting at different ages in the next section and in more depth in subsequent chapters.

TABLE 1.2. Balanced Parenting by Stages of Development

Stage and age	Developmental challenges	Balanced parenting	Resilient child outcomes
Infant (birth–12 months)	• Attachment versus separation	• Responsiveness versus self-care	• Trust (I am loved)
Toddler (1–2 years)	• Agency versus helplessness	• Providing safety versus allowing exploration	• Courage (I can come and go)
Early childhood (3–5 years)	• Initiative versus fearfulness	• Having control versus offering choices	• Character (I am good)
Middle childhood (6–11 years)	• Perseverance versus self-doubt	• Setting limits versus encouraging independence	• Competence (I can do things)
Tweens and young teens (12–15 years)	• Questioning versus confusion	• Setting boundaries versus encouraging autonomy	• Confidence (I am learning who I am; I believe in myself)
Older teens and young adults (16–25 years)	• Identity versus conflicted	• Letting go versus staying involved	• Purpose (I have a plan; I care for myself and others)

Balanced Parenting During Infancy Develops Trust

Balanced parenting during infancy helps babies feel secure and develop the ability to *trust* others. By being responsive to a baby's needs while maintaining their own health and well-being, parents provide babies with the experience of being cared for by healthy, capable adults whose needs are also being met. Balanced parenting avoids extremes. During the first year of life, parents learn how to distinguish cries of distress that need immediate responses from cries of boredom or frustration. Parents learn how to balance meeting their needs and the needs of others in the family with the demands of this new little human who is completely dependent on them for survival. It is not an easy task, but consider the damage that going to either extreme can cause.

The effects of extreme unresponsiveness during infancy were demonstrated by conditions in the Romanian orphanages of the 1990s. Following the overthrow of dictator Nicolae Ceauşescu, human rights workers discovered thousands of infants and young children in orphanages too crowded to provide even basic care. Babies had received only minimal human contact, being swaddled in tight blankets and left in cribs with bottles propped on blankets and towels at feeding time. Researchers have followed these children, some of whom were placed into therapeutic adoptions with caring families. All of them have experienced some difficulties in forming attachments with caregivers, especially those who remained in the orphanages (M. Wade et al., 2020).

At the other extreme are infants of indulgent parents who are never allowed to fuss for more than a few seconds without being picked up, carried, fed, or having a toy waved in their faces as a distraction. In these situations, responsiveness crosses a line into insensitivity, where parents' fears and worries make it difficult for them to tolerate seeing their offspring spend a moment unhappy. When this happens, the baby misses out on the opportunity to learn how to soothe themself by looking around the room, noticing colors, hearing sounds, or just waving their arms in the air. This type of parenting can lead to problems with anxiety and depression as children age.

Balanced Parenting During Toddlerhood Develops Courage

Most parents of 2-year-olds are familiar with the occasional melt-downs and tantrums as toddlers learn to manage this new and powerful experience of having a mind of their own. When parents create safe, child-proofed environments for toddlers to explore rather than punishing them for exploring unsafe settings, children can exert themselves without feeling fearful or helpless. They learn that they can have some control over their world. Resilience is enhanced when parents can successfully manage their own fears and anxieties, learning how to allow the toddler to separate from them to explore while providing a safe environment free from dangerous objects or situations. The toddler develops a sense of personal agency (I can come and go) rather than feeling helpless. *Courage* develops when children see that they can leave the parent and explore another room or part of their space while the parent remains calm as the child toddles away and provides comfort when they return. Toddlers whose parents are too anxious to let them explore a bit on their own prevent them from learning they are still loved and safe when they are on their own.

Balanced Parenting During Early Childhood Develops Character

Around 3 to 5 years of age, most children enter the larger world through playgroups, preschool, or kindergarten. The resilience building block that develops during this stage is *character*. As children begin to interact more regularly with adults, peers, and other children outside of the home and neighborhood, they begin to understand the importance of getting along with others and the need to take the perspectives of others, share one's things and others' attention, and give and receive acts of kindness. As children learn to take the initiative and responsibility for their actions, they begin to develop a sense of goodness or character. Parents can facilitate this by letting go of some of the control and giving children more opportunities to make choices. Preschoolers look to adults to model their behavior and begin to feel proud of themselves for doing the right thing, making good choices, and gaining their parents' and other caregivers' approval. This helps them develop an internal compass of right and wrong, avoiding the anxiety of wondering if they are good or bad. Character is a powerful building block for resilience because it enables children to trust their choices and empathize and connect with others without guilt or fear. Many preschools recognize the foundational importance of the preschool years for the development of character and explicitly teach children about the virtues that promote well-functioning communities and societies and have materials to help parents include them in their conversations at home (see Chapter 4).

Balanced Parenting During Middle Childhood Develops Competence

As children enter the school-age years, their worlds continue to expand, as do pressures to learn and acquire new skills. The balancing act facing parents during middle childhood is helping children learn how to manage new challenges and develop mastery without becoming anxious or overwhelmed and to persist when they don't initially succeed at tasks. Balanced parenting involves granting children opportunities to handle more things on their own while still protecting them from the consequences of failures. Children who learn how to persist in the face of difficult school assignments, who set goals for themselves in sports or their hobbies, and who learn how to work and play with others during middle childhood develop a belief in their *competence*, an important aspect of resilience. This is related to the idea of the "growth mindset" currently being taught in elementary school curriculums. Developmental psychologist Carol Dweck observed thousands of children in classrooms, trying to understand why initial failure prompted some children to try harder and eventually succeed while other children seemed to give up. She discovered that children who blamed their difficulties on their lack of ability were more likely to quit trying because they assumed their abilities were unchangeable or fixed. They had a "fixed mindset." In contrast, children who blamed their difficulties on their inexperience or not trying hard enough, which are changeable qualities, were motivated to persist until they succeeded. Those children have a growth mindset (Dweck, 2017). Developing a growth mindset is now recognized as a valuable characteristic for all of us and is certainly an important aspect of resilience; it is even taught to students at Harvard Business School. Balanced parenting helps children develop this growth mindset by avoiding the extremes of setting expectations that are too high on the one hand or too low on the other and by providing just enough support without solving children's problems or doing all the hard work for them. Believing that "I can do this" allows children to persist when tasks are difficult.

Balanced Parenting During Early Adolescence Develops Confidence

Parenting children on the cusp of adolescence requires allowing them to begin developing a sense of who they are, which may differ from parents' ideas of who they should be. Children between childhood and adolescence, or "tweens," as they are commonly called, and young teens become acutely aware of how they compare with their peers, constantly comparing themselves with others and forming closer attachments to their friends. They begin to question the truth or validity of their parents' teachings and values. This is a normal and important step in developing one's values, but it can create conflict and hurt feelings within families. Balanced parenting recognizes the importance of both the need to separate and identify one's values while also staying connected to family. It sounds like an impossible task, but it can be as simple as making sure that kids know that they must check in at agreed-on times when away from home or parents spending time getting to know their children's friends and their friends' parents. Culture-affirming events and rituals, such as *quinceañeras* or bar and bat mitzvahs, have helped countless generations of parents navigate this delicate process of allowing children to question and explore their values as they move from the innocence of childhood into the larger world. When parents allow children to question and discuss the relative value of family or cultural norms, they help their children develop a more *confident* sense of self.

Balanced Parenting During Late Adolescence and Young Adulthood Develops Purpose

Leaving home is one of the most exciting and difficult accomplishments parents help children achieve. For some youth, it is easier to part when there is a bit of rebellion, and an "I can do this better than you can" attitude helps propel the launch. For others, the transition seems effortless, with an easy move from home to college to apartment with greater financial and emotional independence accompanying each step. Most families will experience something in between, with each child finding their own way to leave the security of home for the thrill of making their way in the world. Balanced parenting looks for ways to help each child find their path, choosing the occupational and life goals that suit them best. Some of these paths will not go as planned, and parents are more and more frequently finding that young adults need longer to prepare for independence than previous generations. The challenge for parents continues to be how to turn over decisions to their almost-grown children, letting them experience the consequences of those decisions while also being available to talk about the lessons learned or help pick up pieces when the consequences are truly painful. We want to prevent our children from suffering, but they learn best when they are allowed to work things out for themselves. It is no easy task to discover one's *purpose* in life, one's partner, or one's place in the world, but that is the task facing our children as they leave our care. Our job at this stage is to be on the sidelines, cheering them on when they succeed, encouraging them when their courage lags, and helping them pick up the pieces and try again when their plans fall apart.

We began this chapter looking in on two parents feeling overwhelmed and worried late one Friday night. But their stories didn't end where we left them.

In the case of our new mom, Emma, just as she was about to reach the tipping point in her fears, her mother texted and asked if she could come and give her a hand in the morning. Emma gladly accepted the offer, even knowing that her mom might make a comment or two about the unfolded laundry or the vegetables becoming science experiments in the refrigerator. Then her partner joined her on the floor after finishing some online work, handed her a cup of chamomile tea, and grabbed a basket of laundry to fold. As suddenly as she had felt despair at ever feeling competent to care for two babies, her heart now soared. True, having twins meant double the laundry (and diapers and feedings and who knows what else to come), but she wasn't alone. Her challenge, she realized, was learning how to rely on others after growing up in a home with a single mom who had trusted no one and done everything herself. It wouldn't be easy, but she could do this!

Across town, our friend Roosevelt jumped when he heard car doors in the driveway. He took a few deep breaths to give his heart a chance to slow down and cool the anger that was already replacing his fear. He was the picture of calm when his two suitably nervous teens came into the kitchen, and he simply asked them, "What happened that you were late?" As his son and daughter talked over themselves with excuses, blaming the game's overtime that they just couldn't leave, the traffic leaving the stadium, the old cell phone that always dies too quickly, the charger that "someone" took out of the car and didn't replace, he looked at them both and realized what good kids they were. He surprised them both by saying that there was no real harm done except for a few new gray hairs on their old father's head and asked them what they could do to make sure it didn't happen again. He saw the relief wash over them as they began to throw out ideas to prevent a reoccurrence. And he realized that they were going to be okay. If staying out of trouble and emotionally connected to their dad was this important to them, he believed they would be able to figure out the next few years one day and one conversation at a time.

ACTIVITY: SETTING YOUR DESTINATION

Being a balanced parent requires us to be aware of our child-rearing goals and to be cooperative and communicative when sharing those goals with partners and other caregivers. Mothers, fathers, grandparents, and other caregivers often have different priorities for managing children's competing developmental needs. For example, one parent may come from a family that valued obedience, with strict limits and limited freedom, while the other parent may have grown up in a family that valued independence, with considerable autonomy and tolerance. These differences in expectations can create conflicts between parents and other caregivers if they do not talk about their values and goals for their children. In fact, when we try to avoid conflict, we are likely to create more conflict because underlying assumptions and values are left unspoken. Gaining experience in talking about different priorities and developing the ability to acknowledge the importance of different perspectives is an important—even essential—component of developing resilience as parents and promoting resilience in children.

If we were with colleagues talking about our goals for a major project that would require the next 20-plus years of our lives to complete, we would probably be encouraged to sit down and come up with a statement of values, our mission, and how we will know whether we are succeeding. We may have rolled our eyes a time or two when we were asked to attend meetings or retreats to come up with these statements, but we can't deny the importance of getting clear about our goals and milestones in developing successful projects. We think it is even more important when our "product" is a human being than when it is a new product line or program! The clearer we are about our intentions, the more focused our personal work will be.

We encourage you to spend some time now thinking about what qualities you value most in yourself and others. We believe that we help our children and ourselves become more resilient when we are aware and intentional about the qualities we want our children to develop and when we routinely model and label those values in everyday life.

We have included a list of values that many parents want their children to develop, adapted from the work of Dr. Catherine Tamis-LeMonda and colleagues (2008) at New York University. We invite you to think and talk about your values with your partner and others who care for your children. As you have these conversations, be open to the importance of values that others prioritize. These conversations will be helpful with the balancing acts that make up everyday decisions and responses to children's behavior.

In Chapter 4, when we focus on the development of children's overall character, we talk more explicitly about the strategies parents can use to help their children develop these values and other strengths that will help them throughout their lives.

1. Read through the list of values below. Think about what values you would like to see in your children as they grow up. Write down the top three for each of your children.

    _____

    _____

    _____

    Curiosity
    Determination
    Friendliness
    Helpfulness
    Honesty
    Kindness
    Loyalty
    Obedience
    Respect
    Self-discipline

2. If you are raising your children with a spouse or other parenting partner, invite them to go through and write down their most important values. How do your values overlap or differ?

    _____

    _____

3. Are there other values not on this list that you think are important for your child to have?

    _____

    _____

    _____

Take time to discuss your values with your partner, especially if they differ. Later in this book, we provide a framework for having conversations when points of view differ. Feel free to skip ahead and read about tips for having these crucial conversations at the end of Chapter 7 if you disagree about values for your children.

RESOURCES

General Parenting

Cline, F., & Fay, J. (2020). *Parenting with love and logic*. NavPress.

Faber, A., & Mazlish, E. (2012). *How to talk so kids will listen & listen so kids will talk*. Simon & Schuster.

Ginott, H. G. (2009). *Between parent and child*. Harmony.

Siegel, D. J., & Bryson, T. P. (2011). *The whole-brain child: 12 revolutionary strategies to nurture your child's developing mind*. Delacorte Press.

Steinberg, L. D. (2005). *The ten basic principles of good parenting*. Simon & Schuster.

A blog with science-based advice for parents: https://childandfamilyblog.com

CHAPTER 2

ACEs AND PACEs: HOW ADVERSE AND PROTECTIVE EXPERIENCES AFFECT YOU AND YOUR CHILD

It was 1936 in San Angelo, Texas. The nation was in the depths of the Great Depression, and West Texas was enduring the worst of the dust bowl. Jennifer's father was 5 years old, the middle child of seven children ranging from 11 months to 15 years, when his mother went into the hospital for gall bladder surgery. His older sister wrote about what happened next in her memoirs: "Mother had the surgery, and it was successful. But about 10 days after surgery, she developed pneumonia and died a few days later. That was before antibiotics, so pneumonia was deadly then. She was 37 years of age. I can remember the empty, lost feeling I had at 12 years. Daddy didn't keep us together long after mother died. I don't know why, but he just could not seem to take responsibility. He put the four little boys in an orphanage and said they could be adopted. It is hard to sit here and write these things down; I've never felt so sad, so unloved and unwanted—I can't find words to say how I felt" (W. M. H. Copeland, personal communication, November 1999).

One of their mother's friends went to the orphanage, picked up the four little boys, took them off the adoption list, and kept them for a short time. The teenage son joined the air force, and the two teenage girls lived with an aunt. The four little Hays boys, as they became known (see Figure 2.1), spent the next 3 years in foster homes, sometimes

FIGURE 2.1. The Four Hays Boys

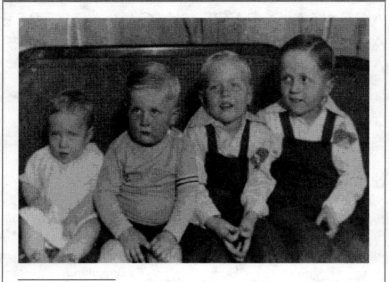

Jennifer's father Curtis (5), far right, and his younger brothers from left to right, Farrell (1), John (2), and Bob (4), on the day of their mother's funeral.

two together but usually alone, sometimes with relatives, and sometimes with strangers. One night after moving to a new place, 4-year-old Bob had a dream that stayed with him for the rest of his life. In his dream, he got mad and stomped his foot on the front porch. At that instant, everything around him exploded, and he was alone in the world.

After 3 years of moving about, the four little boys were reunited. A social worker had placed their names on the waiting list for a new children's home being built 90 miles away in Abilene, Texas. On a sunny November day in 1939, the Hays boys walked through the big double doors into the Hendrick Home for Children. They moved into rooms on the "little boys' floor," where they met Fanny Rae Durham, a woman who would care for them until they left the home. Later, she would move upstairs with them to the "big boys' floor," and Jennifer knew her as grand mommy. "The Home," as it is still affectionately known, was the legacy of Ida and Tom Hendrick, who used their wealth to create a truly progressive institution then and now. The caregivers and resources at the Hendrick Home for Children were some of the reasons Jennifer's father and his brothers grew up to become good citizens, husbands, and fathers.

The Hays boys were finally given the stability and resources they needed to be resilient, but the adversity they experienced as children took a toll on them. By midlife, each of them had developed diabetes, high blood pressure, and heart disease. Now, their children and grandchildren wonder about the effects of their fathers' early adversity on their own health. They are right to wonder because there is evidence that the damaging effects of childhood adversity can be passed from one generation to the next. One of the reasons we wrote this book was to help families break the cycles of adversity that continue to reverberate throughout their histories.

In this chapter, we describe the ways that adverse childhood experiences (ACEs) and other types of trauma and stress can get "under the skin," causing lifelong health problems and other difficulties. Importantly, we also describe how protective and compensatory experiences (PACEs) can lessen the effects of ACEs and promote healing. At the end of the chapter, we invite you to complete the ACEs and PACEs surveys and think about how your childhood adverse and protective experiences may have shaped your development.

WHAT ARE ACEs?

The negative effects of abuse, neglect, or growing up in a home with domestic violence, alcohol or substance abuse, and other detrimental conditions have long been recognized. What was not fully understood was the effect of these experiences when they occur in combination, as many of them do. This changed when Dr. Vince Felitti, who directed the preventive medicine clinic for the Kaiser Foundation Health Plan in San Diego, and Dr. Robert Anda, a researcher at the Centers for Disease Control and Prevention, began asking thousands of adult Kaiser patients about their ACEs (see Table 2.1 and Figure 2.2) and linked their ACEs with their health problems and health-harming behaviors. Their results, first published in 1998, stunned Drs. Felitti and Anda. First, no one had ever revealed just how widespread childhood trauma and adversity

TABLE 2.1. Percentage of Adverse Childhood Experiences (ACEs) in the Original ACEs Study

Type of ACE	Total %
Physical abuse	28
Parent substance abuse	27
Divorce/separation	23
Sexual abuse	20
Parent mental illness	19
Emotional neglect	15
Domestic violence	13
Emotional abuse	11
Physical neglect	10
Parent incarcerated	5

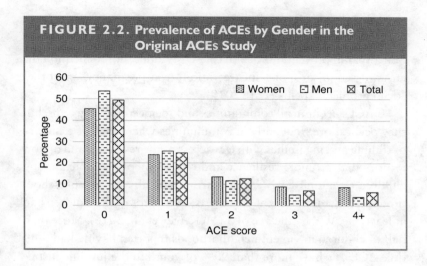

FIGURE 2.2. Prevalence of ACEs by Gender in the Original ACEs Study

are in our society. In this largely middle-class, well-insured group of adults, nearly two thirds reported having one or more of the 10 ACEs.

More than one quarter of the Kaiser patients reported physical abuse, and more than one quarter reported that a parent had drug or alcohol problems. They also found that most people who had one ACE also had at least one additional ACE because different types of adversities tend to co-occur. Most importantly, ACEs had a cumulative, or "dose–response," effect. In other words, as the number of ACEs increased, so did the risk of serious physical and mental health problems, including heart disease, cancer, lung disease, autoimmune disorders, and depression. ACEs also predicted health-harming behaviors, including smoking, misuse of alcohol and other drugs, early and unprotected sexual activity, and suicide attempts (Anda et al., 2006; Felitti et al., 1998).

Since the first ACEs publication in 1998, thousands of papers from all over the world have supported these findings, allowing us to state without a doubt that ACEs are both global and destructive. ACEs have been estimated to cost North America at least $748 billion a year in preventable health care costs alone, not to mention the costs of school dropout, incarceration, teen pregnancy, and other social problems (Bellis et al., 2019).

ACEs occur in all communities and socioeconomic groups, but they occur more frequently in communities where there is a history of trauma and in families with less access to the resources and opportunities that promote resilience and recovery. For example, among children attending Early Head Start, a federally funded preschool program for children living in poverty, two thirds of the children had at least one ACE by the age of 5 (McKelvey et al., 2016). More than half of children in violent neighborhoods reported having had multiple ACEs, as have more than 90% of youth in the juvenile justice system (Baglivio et al., 2014; R. Wade et al., 2014).

Research conducted since the original study has made us aware that other types of adverse childhood experiences are not included in the original ACEs questionnaire. These include bullying, discrimination, neighborhood violence, and being a refugee of war or other disasters. Certainly, if events or situations are intense, chronic, or have other negative consequences on children's well-being, they are likely to have negative long-term consequences on children's development and later health. As you think about ACEs in your own life or the lives of those close to you, do not discount events or situations that were traumatic just because they are not listed on the original ACEs questionnaire.

EFFECTS OF ACEs ON THE BODY AND BRAIN

We all know that stress can affect our health. Magazines and other media are full of advice on how to reduce our stress so that we can sleep better, feel better, and avoid illness by boosting our immune systems. Imagine you are driving one afternoon on a four-lane highway when the car coming toward you suddenly veers across the yellow lines into your lane, heading straight at you. You immediately swerve into the lane to your right without even checking to see if another car is in that lane. Fortunately, that lane was empty, and the driver of the oncoming car recognizes their mistake and goes back to their lane, and a potentially fatal crash is avoided. As you read this, you can almost feel your body reacting if you allow yourself to picture this scenario. Your heart rate speeds up, your rate of breathing increases, your skin tingles as blood races to your hands, arms, legs, and feet, and your body stops doing many other things (like digesting your lunch) while it produces the tiny signaling proteins and hormones that will ensure your immediate survival in the face of danger. Our bodies do this because our ancestors were able to respond with extraordinary strength and agility when they encountered saber tooth tigers, and they passed those survival skills down to us through our genes. Those whose bodies were less responsive to danger did not live as long and were less likely to pass their genes to subsequent generations.

You have probably heard this physical response to perceived danger referred to as the *fight–flight–freeze response*. This response is obviously adaptive because it ensures that the body and brain work seamlessly together to mount an orchestrated response to perceived threats to survival. The problem occurs when those perceived threats are frequent or chronic, when our bodies are constantly exposed to cortisol and other stress hormones produced in response to those perceived threats. As helpful as these physical reactions are for immediate survival, they can be toxic to cells and organs over the long term. And as damaging as stress hormones are for adults, their effects on children's developing cells, organs, and brains are even more harmful.

When children are exposed to repeated events and situations that elicit the fight–flight–freeze response, their bodies can respond in several ways. One response is to be hypervigilant. In our highway example, imagine that every few miles, someone from the oncoming traffic lane crosses into our lane. Assuming that you don't have the option to go off the road and wait for a helicopter to take you to your destination, you have no option but to proceed carefully, scanning for oncoming cars and staying in a constant state of hyperarousal. This is the situation when children's living situations involve abuse, neglect, or other types of threats to their safety. The child's body and brain unconsciously adapt to ACEs by staying in a super alert, hypervigilant state. At the other extreme, some children adapt to constant stress by shutting off their alarm systems, becoming hypo-vigilant or underresponsive, shutting out external cues. While it can be adaptive in the short term not to get upset every time someone in the household is violent or verbally abusive, it can have the long-term effect of making it difficult to pay attention to others' cues or be responsive to real dangers. It may even cause children to seek extreme thrills to feel anything at all.

Another consequence of chronic exposure to stress in child-hood is its effect on inflammation and the immune system. Stress triggers inflammation because when our ancestors were running from those saber tooth tigers in our prehistoric past, their survival depended on being able to repair injuries sustained during those encounters. The connection between stress and inflammation still exists. Inflammation helps us recover from injuries and disease in the short term (just like that cortisone shot you got to help you recover from that case of poison ivy), but it has damaging effects on cells and tissues over time (which is why they limit the number of shots you can have). There is a balance between having an inflammatory response to an acute injury or disease and maintaining a healthy immune system over time.

In some situations, adaptations to stress can become some-what permanent as the body learns to survive in extreme conditions.

Researchers have found changes in the genes of some individuals who have experienced trauma or adversity, a process called *epigenesis*. For example, genes that help the body get rid of stress hormones may be turned off or reduced in quantity, making it more likely that the stress hormones continue to circulate in the body long after the perceived or actual threat has passed. This is like reprogramming the sensor of a car alarm to go off when someone walks by, rather than when someone tries to force open the door, and to stay on even when no further threat is sensed. While this may be advantageous in keeping the child ready to respond quickly when threats are constant, it also prevents their body from returning to the relaxed, receptive, and calm state in which learning occurs, relationships are formed, and physical recovery from stress occurs.

When children experience significant episodes of stress from abuse, neglect, and family dysfunction, the effects can be cumulative and have enduring effects on their ability to pay attention, control their emotions and behavior, and form stable relationships with others. Stress and adversity may also change children's brain development, shaping how they think, learn, and remember (see Figure 2.3).

In this way, ACEs and other traumatic events have other detrimental effects. If these problems are not addressed when they occur, children may do poorly in school, have trouble making friends, and struggle to acquire the knowledge and skills they need to enjoy a productive and meaningful life. Instead of entering the world with confidence and positive expectations, youth from abusive, neglectful, and dysfunctional families often feel ill prepared to enter adult life. They may feel most comfortable with similarly unhappy and angry youth, forming attachments with others who are lacking in emotional and social skills. They may try to find a release from negative thoughts and emotions through alcohol or drugs, which further deteriorates their ability to experience real

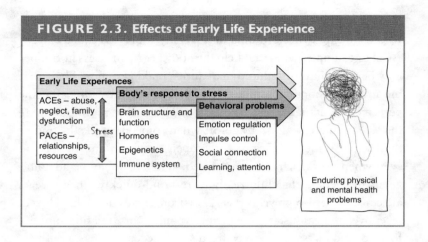

FIGURE 2.3. Effects of Early Life Experience

joy, connect genuinely with others, and find their purpose in life. In short, ACEs can be devastating to development and long-term well-being.

However, ACEs do not always destroy one's life. In fact, we know many joyful, talented, and inspiring individuals who experienced significant adversities as children. When we talked with them about their childhoods, we learned that there were always reasons why they were able to survive and even thrive. Sometimes there were many reasons for their resilience in the face of adversity. These reasons almost always included having loving and helpful people in their lives—a grandmother, teacher, or best friend—or having access to resources—going to a good school, having an engaging hobby, being involved in sports. When we reviewed decades of research on what distinguished children who were resilient from their peers who were not, we made our list of PACEs—10 protective and compensatory experiences that help children do well in spite of adversity.

PACEs: THE ANTIDOTE TO ACEs

If you had discovered that you had taken a bite of a poisonous apple and someone offered you the antidote, you would take it without asking questions. After you take it and the danger passes, you might be curious about how the antidote managed to neutralize or reduce the effects of the poison. That is how we think about the effects of the 10 PACEs. We know that PACEs can reduce the toxic stress caused by ACEs and help adults recover from childhood adversity. We know this because we have read hundreds of research studies that identified the aspects of resilient children's environments, children who were able to survive and thrive as adults in spite of traumatic and difficult childhood circumstances. In fact, Dr. Ann Masten (2015), a well-known psychologist at the University of Minnesota, calls this phenomenon "ordinary magic." Her decades of research on resilience showed that families and communities have created ways over time to ensure that their members are able to survive and thrive in the face of adversity. We have also done our own research. We wondered whether PACEs had the same cumulative dose–response effect as ACEs. The answer is an emphatic yes! The more protective experiences, the better. We and others have found that children become resilient when they have both positive and nurturing relationships and enriching environments (Morris et al., 2021).

Before we describe each of the PACEs, we want to be clear about what we mean by the word *resilient*. We hear this word used a lot, particularly since the COVID pandemic, and not everyone uses it the same way. Resilience is often thought of as "bouncing back" from some traumatic or difficult experience. While the notion of bouncing back is appealing, it is not completely accurate because no one is ever exactly the same after encountering trauma or adversity. Experiences change us—all our experiences, both positive and negative. Our brain records each new experience, creating new synapses and memory stores—even if we don't consciously remember the experience. As we previously discussed, our DNA may even change because genetic material may be altered to better prepare us for encountering that experience again. Depending on the intensity or frequency of exposure to adversity, our conscious attitudes and expectations about the world and responses to others may change.

Rather than thinking of resilience as bouncing back from adversity, we believe that resilience is a process of continually moving forward—learning, growing, gaining wisdom and perspective. This is possible when we have sufficient love, support, opportunities, and resources to develop even in the face of adversity. Providing children with the relationships and the means to protect and compensate for adversity in childhood is one of the most powerful tools available to parents. While we want to protect children from trauma and unnecessary hardship, we know we are not always with them and cannot always provide that protection. So, we build into our everyday routines the opportunities for them to feel safe and loved and begin developing skills and abilities. Then when adversities occur, as they will, they have the habits, attitudes, and perspectives to cope. We use the word *compensate* because these positive experiences can often balance or counteract adversity, helping to offset the negative experiences with pleasant recollections and examples of practices to emulate in the future.

We also note that PACEs work for adults as well as children. When we provide children exposed to ACEs with these protective and compensating experiences, we help them build resilience by offsetting the negative with the positive and increasing their internal and external resources to cope with adversity. With adults, PACEs provide the opportunities to recover from past ACEs, creating the relationships and structure to support growth, insight, new habits, and coping strategies. When parents begin implementing PACEs for themselves as well as with their children, real transformation can happen, creating homes of harmony, love, stability, and joy.

10 PACEs THAT PROTECT AND STRENGTHEN YOUR CHILD

PACEs are aspects of the physical, social, and emotional environments that build resilience in children and adults. When researchers first tried to understand how some children became resilient after adversity, they focused on the characteristics of the children themselves. They noted that resilient children tended to be smarter, outgoing, more physically attractive, and good at sports or other socially valued skills. These findings make sense to us because we know that teachers and other adults are likely to invest more time and overlook more behavior problems in children they perceive as attractive, intelligent, or gifted in some way. But these are not qualities that are easily modified or possessed by all children. What about the resilient children who did not have these qualities? What was in the lives of these children that made a difference? We discovered that 10 aspects of children's lives increased resilience.

Ten years ago, we knew that each PACE had been found to be linked to being resilient, but we did not know if PACEs would have a cumulative, or dose–response, effect. So we asked hundreds of adults to recall which of these 10 experiences they remembered having, as well as what ACEs they had. Then we analyzed whether the total number of PACEs affected their well-being and their attitudes about parenting. We found that the number of PACEs was positively related to adult well-being and parenting attitudes, especially for adults who had high ACE scores (Morris et al., 2021). We continue to do research on PACEs, and we are confident that we know enough now to advocate that everyone—especially parents who have had ACEs or whose children have ACEs—will benefit by making these 10 PACEs part of their lives.

Table 2.2 lists each of the 10 PACEs and briefly outlines how they are expressed at each major stage of life from birth to adulthood. The five relationship PACEs are love, guidance, friendship,

TABLE 2.2. Protective and Compensatory Experiences (PACEs) From Birth to Adulthood

	Birth to 5	Middle childhood	Adolescence	Adulthood
Love				
	• Nurturing and responsive care from parent or caregiver	• Love from parent or caregiver not used as reward or punishment	• Strong, positive relationships with parents, allowing more independence	• Being loved and cared for by a partner or close friend
Guidance				
	• Time spent with nurturing adults outside of immediate family	• Supportive teachers or other caring adults	• Opportunities for guidance from trusted adults	• Positive relationships with older, wiser adults
Friendship				
	• One-on-one play with peers and siblings	• Spending time with one or two best friends from school, family, or neighborhood	• Continuation of childhood friendships and addition of new ones as interests change	• Keeping cherished friends and making new friends at each stage of life

Affiliation

• Group play and interactions with adult supervision	• Social groups and clubs through school, interests, or neighborhood	• Expanded network of associations based on interests, aspirations	• Membership in groups for personal and professional support and benefit

Benevolence

• Observing and practicing empathy and caring for others	• Being helpful at home, school, neighborhood	• Taking part in volunteer groups and activities	• Being actively engaged in community volunteering and altruistic actions

Stability

• Regular, predictable schedule for meeting physical and emotional needs	• Consistent times, routines, and rituals to accomplish daily tasks pleasantly	• Reasonable changes in routines to allow more self-regulation	• Structured but flexible routines and rituals that support goals and values

Comfort

• Food, clothing, and hygienic, safe, and uncluttered home	• Involvement and cooperation in chores to keep a healthy home	• Increased responsibility for ensuring healthy living conditions	• Intentional actions to ensure safe, healthy, and orderly household

(continues)

TABLE 2.2. Protective and Compensatory Experiences (PACEs) From Birth to Adulthood (Continued)

Knowledge		
• Opportunities to learn through talking, reading, unstructured play, and being outdoors	• Schools and other settings that provide resources for cognitive and social-emotional development	• Educational resources to identify and develop skills and abilities needed for adult life	• Resources to increase knowledge and skills and grow as a person, partner, parent, member of society
Movement		
• Regular active and outdoor play	• Instruction and time to develop physical skills and sporting interests	• Time and opportunity to be physically active individually or in organized groups	• Regular physical activity to stay healthy and strong throughout adulthood
Recreation		
• Resources readily available to play creatively	• Opportunities and materials to develop creative or other talents and interests	• Time and resources for self-motivated development of creative hobbies	• Opportunities to cultivate engaging and relaxing hobbies and pastimes

affiliation, and benevolence, and the five resource PACEs are stability, comfort, knowledge, movement, and recreation. Each of these is described in Table 2.2 and discussed with more detail and examples in the chapters to follow.

PACE 1: Love

Of all the PACEs studied by researchers across the world, having a parent's or other caregiver's unconditional love is by far the most beneficial and powerful protective experience a child can have. All of us, especially young children who are dependent on others for their survival as well as their growth and development, need the security that comes from feeling loved unconditionally. What do we mean by *unconditionally*? We mean that while you may feel angry or disappointed at your child's behavior, you don't stop loving or caring for them and make them feel that your love will be withdrawn if their actions do not meet your expectations. In fact, your children need to hear that you will always love them, even if you are upset with them.

During infancy and early childhood, unconditional love is transmitted by feeding, changing, bathing, holding, and comforting them and by creating a sort of zone of safety from which they can begin to explore their world in wider and wider circles. For older children, unconditional love is expressed by not using love as a reward or punishment and by seeing the good in them even as they struggle with meeting the growing expectations of school and peers.

All children will test the bounds of unconditional love at times; otherwise, how would they know it is truly unconditional? Especially in adolescence, our offspring will stretch parental love to the limits as they seek their independence and overestimate their readiness to be free of adult rules and supervision. Unconditional love can be especially powerful then because it lets teens know that their parents are their best option when they face situations they can't handle, such as when they need a ride home when they've disobeyed the rules and gone to a party and had too much to drink. Unconditional love is still important in adulthood and provides a solid foundation to build a family and nurture children. Learning to love unconditionally and that one deserves unconditional love is a big step in recovering from childhood trauma.

PACE 2: Guidance

Having support and assistance from trustworthy adults outside of one's family is an important aspect of recovering from childhood adversity. When one's family lacks the ability to provide children and youth with the emotional support or practical advice to develop their potential and move toward their aspirations, having outside mentors can be life changing. A trustworthy adult provides support, advice, and comfort when parents are not available or helpful. Grandparents are also a source of unconditional love for babies and young children, along with aunts, uncles, and other extended family members. They also provide older children and teens with a safe adult with whom they can share their frustrations. They can ask questions they are uncomfortable asking their parents, learn to solve problems, and observe different ways of behaving as an adult.

We have heard many resilient adults talk about the importance of a teacher who first recognized their worth as a human being, giving them the confidence to fit in with their peers, do well in school, and dare to dream of a better future. As adults, it is common to have mentors in our jobs or professional lives, relying on more experienced workers to help us learn the ropes or advance our careers. This same idea is helpful when applied to partnering, parenting, and developing our relationship skills. Jennifer's brother Jeff summoned the courage to ask a well-respected man in his community to mentor him as a father after a divorce left Jeff raising four children on his own. This man was so active in his family and community that the only time he had available was at 11 p.m., so Jeff drove an hour each way once a month to get this sage man's advice on being a good father. The life-altering advice and wisdom given to Jeff in those late-night conversations 20 years ago continue to influence everyone in Jeff's extended family today.

PACE 3: Friendship

Having a best friend is an important aspect of developing socially and emotionally across all stages of childhood and adolescence. Even during infancy and early childhood, children learn from having opportunities to play with other children their age, getting their first glimpse of the social world of taking turns, sharing objects, and not hurting others when angry. These lessons are much easier to learn in the context of a favorite playmate demanding a turn on the swing than listening to a parent giving a lecture on sharing. And there is nothing more delightful than hearing two toddlers laughing hilariously over some shared discovery or private joke. In middle childhood, children are protected from peer rejection and bullying when they have a best friend. With a best friend, they have another source of support and acceptance from outside the family, can try out new skills, and learn about different patterns and routines of other families. During adolescence, best friends continue to serve a protective role for children and youth who have experienced ACEs.

Best friends are not only a source of support but can also provide access to other adults and resources necessary for successfully entering adulthood. It is normal for best friends to change as one's interests change, and by adulthood, it is possible to have several "best" friends. For example, you may have one in the neighborhood, one or two from childhood, one from work, and one from the parents of your children's friends. Recognizing the value of friends is important and worth the effort to make time to spend together.

Without good friends, life can be lonely, and loneliness is a threat not only to resilience but also to health and life itself.

PACE 4: Affiliation

Just as having a best friend promotes resilience and well-being in childhood, being part of a large social group is also protective against the effects of ACEs. Going to preschool provides toddlers and young children with opportunities to interact with and learn from other children in a safe and structured place. As children become school-age, they benefit from membership in youth organizations and clubs where they can gain a sense of belonging in the community, explore their identity, and have fun doing activities with other children their age. Adolescence is a time of focused activities when teens gravitate toward groups of others who share their interests and hobbies. Being part of scouts, faith-based youth groups, music groups (choir, orchestra, band), or other interest-driven groups can help children and youth make friends and feel connected, especially if they have recently moved to a new school or neighborhood.

Parents benefit when they spend the time and effort to support their children's social groups and benefit from their own membership in both personally and vocationally supportive groups and associations. There are so many demands on parents' time in today's world that it may seem frivolous or unimportant to make time for supportive social groups, such as a book club, but they are vital at every age for staying connected with one's community, and they help maintain mental health and build lifelong resilience.

PACE 5: Benevolence

One way to be positively connected with one's community is by volunteering. Being involved in community volunteering events and activities helps children learn about the needs of others. It helps develop empathy, altruism, and perspective taking. It encourages children to develop a sense of gratitude for what they have, as they recognize that there are others with less—poor health, lack of food, or inadequate housing. Even very young children can be involved in observing and helping parents engage in altruistic or humanitarian efforts. These can be actions as simple as asking young children to select items to donate to the food pantry when you are grocery shopping; taking turns planting, watering, or weeding at the local school garden (or helping other parents start one); or supporting your teen's efforts to raise money or accompany local groups providing disaster relief in nearby areas. When children volunteer with their parents, both parents and children benefit from the experience of helping others and feel more connected to their community.

PACE 6: Stability

Children, as well as adults, are more likely to feel secure and calm when the world around them is orderly, predictable, and fair. When expectations are clear and rules are consistently applied, children actually have more freedom to act because they know the limits on their behavior. Imagine a dog with an electric fence around the yard to keep them from straying away and getting lost. Once they have learned where the boundaries are, they are free to roam and play within the safe space. But if the electric fence is one day here and one day there, they are less likely to feel free to play. As babies learn to walk and explore their space, it may be necessary to create physical boundaries within which dangerous objects and conditions are childproofed. As they get older, parents need to be clear about the household rules and expectations—how far children can go on their own, how long they can play on their tablet or watch children's programs, for example.

Predictable routines also create a sense of safety. Having bath and bedtime routines helps children know what to expect and prevents nightly negotiations or arguments. Sleep is vitally important at all stages of development, so having good bedtime routines helps everyone. Parents can prepare their adolescents for eventual adult independence by deciding together about rules to keep them safe while allowing more independence. For example, what time are they expected to be home on weekend and school nights? How often should they check in when they are out with friends? Teens are more likely to tolerate their parents monitoring their activities when they have had a say in creating the rules and understand the reasons for them. Of course, parents also benefit from setting up family routines and being consistent in their behavior, particularly if they did not grow up in well-regulated and orderly families. Chaos and unpredictability breed uncertainty, anxiety, and mistrust and work against creating resilience throughout life.

PACE 7: Comfort

Maybe you remember hearing about Maslow's hierarchy of needs, which states that before you can develop your talents and potential, your basic needs must be met first: food, clothing, and safe shelter. It almost goes without saying that for children to develop into joyous, confident, capable people, they need to have clean and safe places to live, clean clothes, and adequate nutritious foods, but there are many children for whom these basic needs go unmet. They do not live with the basic elements to promote the comfort to heal so that they can grow and learn. Instead, their focus must be on survival. Many communities have created organizations and policies to help parents who find themselves in dire straits to meet these needs, but going without food, diapers, clothing, and shelter, even temporarily, is distressing to parents and harmful to children. In addition, children who live in homes that are cluttered and disorganized have worse outcomes than their peers, even when income and other resources are the same.

Children benefit from being active participants in keeping the home uncluttered and clean. Starting with toddlers and preschoolers, children can help set the table, make sure that pets have water and food, and put away their toys after playing with them. As children develop, they can be involved in meal preparation, fold and put away laundry, sweep, dust, and vacuum as part of daily and weekly family routines. After a lecture on the health danger of eating too much fast food, Jennifer once heard a college student ask the instructor how he could eat meals at home when his mother wasn't there to prepare them. He was completely unaware of the steps involved in making a sandwich. Resilient and capable adults know how to prepare simple and healthy meals, maintain a clean and organized home, and care for their material possessions.

PACE 8: Knowledge

We believe that having opportunities to acquire knowledge and learn skills is crucial for building resilience and is, in fact, a hallmark of a well-lived life. Just as humans are programmed to connect with others, we are born wired to learn. Babies initially acquire knowledge through their senses—eyes, ears, nose, hands, and mouth. Parents may not realize it, but they are their children's first teachers. Your children watch and learn from the expressions on your face, what you do, and what you say. Young children need opportunities to view the world from a safe vantage point, to play and interact with physical objects and other children. When young children whose families live in poverty attend quality early childhood programs such as Early Head Start, they are much less likely as adolescents to drop out of high school, get involved with gangs or criminal activity, or have an unplanned pregnancy. In fact, early childhood education has been found to provide a 13% per year return on investment (https://Heckmanequation.org).

While learning is clearly important during the critical periods of infancy and early childhood, it continues to be important for older children and adolescents. Good schools provide children with the resources and teachers to help them learn a variety of subjects and skills. There is a strong link between attending quality schools and later life success and happiness, especially when children have been exposed to ACEs and other types of traumas. Resilient adults are also always learning. Understanding the world and oneself is not something accomplished overnight. Indeed, it is a lifelong process. When we acknowledge that we still have much to learn, we become open to new perspectives, gain new knowledge, make unexpected discoveries, and become better able to solve problems and navigate new experiences. Not only do we become more resilient but we also become better parents, partners, and people.

PACE 9: Movement

Being physically active increases resilience in several ways. First, physical activity increases brain activity. We now know that physical activity increases the production of hormones that help the brain create new connections between neurons, connections that form the basis for learning and memory. Second, physical activity keeps our bodies healthy by improving heart health, circulation, flexibility, and strength. Third, physical activity is one way the body can discharge stress and eliminate the toxic chemicals created by the fight–flight–freeze response to threatening situations. Physical activity has been found to be an effective strategy for treating depression—more effective than medication alone in randomized clinical trials. Finally, many types of physical activity can also be a source of social connection and protection from harmful health behaviors. Teens who have athletic goals and interests are less likely to use tobacco or illicit drugs or drink alcohol because these behaviors are incompatible with being successful in their sport. Sports also help children learn to set and work toward goals, recover from failures, and celebrate successes. Family outings that include biking, hiking, or other physical activities are great ways for adults and children to enjoy the health benefits of exercise while having fun together.

PACE 10: Recreation

Speaking of having fun, children who have opportunities to develop and enjoy creative and engaging leisure activities are more likely to be resilient. In our competitive and fast-paced world, the importance of spending time on recreational activities is often disregarded. This can be particularly hard for families struggling to make ends meet, but it is still worth the effort to find time and opportunities to enjoy hobbies. Hobbies and recreation provide outlets for creative expression and ways to explore ourselves and the world around us. Reading, drawing, playing the guitar, playing chess, cooking, and engaging in other hobbies is absorbing and challenging. Hobbies can motivate children to persevere toward mastery and excellence because they are having fun in the process, at least most of the time. When children have the opportunity to develop their strengths and pursue their interests and talents, they also feel a sense of competence and justifiable pride in their accomplishments.

Hobbies promote resilience in adolescents and adults, providing an outlet for them to recover a sense of self-worth as individuals, develop self-confidence, and make social connections with others who share their interests. Some hobbies, such as gardening, dancing, and hiking, also help keep us in shape. In fact, adults with active hobbies are less likely to experience stress and depression, and they sleep better. For those who think they don't have time for a hobby, remember that hobbies can also boost one's career; many employers make a point to look for people who have outside interests that they pursue with passion, as do colleges and universities when they are admitting students. Parents who support their children's pursuit of their interests and passions are helping them become resilient in ways they may never have imagined.

PACEs AND BALANCED PARENTING

In combination, balanced parenting and PACEs can break the cycle of adversity that may have existed for generations. In future chapters, we share more specific ways to use balanced parenting strategies and PACEs at each stage of your child's development. As parents, we develop skills that build resilience through practice. Then we are prepared to help our children become resilient through our example and the environment we create that supports the development of their ability to adapt positively to adversity whenever it occurs.

We hope that after this brief description of PACEs, you are beginning to see how they fit into an overall way of being a balanced parent. It may seem overwhelming to think about implementing all these PACEs for you and your child. But go slow. Add one at a time, beginning with the ones that add the most joy and calm to your lives. Remember that PACEs not only promote resilience but they also support the essential responsibilities of being a parent: providing love, meeting basic needs, and giving children opportunities to develop physically, mentally, socially, and emotionally. Our parenting road map is almost complete. Now for the journey itself.

ACTIVITY: YOU ARE HERE

In the last chapter, we talked about knowing where you want to go on your parenting journey and recognizing the values that guide your path. The next important step in a successful journey is knowing your starting point. We recommend thinking about your ACEs and PACEs. This allows you to become more aware of how your childhood experiences may influence your parenting.

On the next few pages, you will find the ACEs and PACEs questionnaires. Feel free to copy these pages if you want to have several copies, or go to our website at https://www.acesandpaces. com/measures.html for downloadable copies. For both the ACEs and the PACEs questionnaires, feel free to list any additional items that served as either adverse or protective experiences during your childhood. For example, bullying, discrimination, or the death of a parent can be aversive experiences. Conversely, other protective experiences can include having the devoted love of a pet or having a spiritual faith that provides meaning in the face of adversity.

As you fill out the ACEs questionnaire, you may find yourself experiencing memories and feelings that you have not allowed yourself to feel in the past. Please contact local mental health hotlines or behavioral health services if you need to talk with someone (see the Resources section at the end of the chapter). Many people are available to help you deal with these feelings. Repressing them is only a short-term strategy, useful only until you have the strength or the support to allow them to surface and be attended to. Most people find that telling their ACEs story to themselves or someone else is the first step in healing and recovering from trauma. We are the creators of our life stories. While we did not create all our experiences, we have control over our responses. We can be the hero of the story and not the victim just by realizing that we are still alive, we are strong, and we are actively seeking and learning how to survive and thrive. By filling out the PACEs questionnaire, we remind ourselves of the other part of our childhood story, identify sources of happiness and support in our lives, and generate ideas for future avenues of growth and joy.

Adverse Childhood Experiences (ACEs)

While you were growing up, during your first 18 years of life:

1. Did a parent or other adult in the household often or very often:

   Swear at you, insult you, put you down, or humiliate you **OR** act in a way that made you afraid that you might be physically hurt?   YES   NO

2. Did a parent or other adult in the household often or very often:

   Push, grab, slap, or throw something at you **OR** hit you so hard that you had marks or were injured?   YES   NO

3. Did an adult or person at least 5 years older than you ever:

   Touch or fondle you or have you touch their body in a sexual way **OR** attempt or actually have oral, anal, or vaginal intercourse with you?   YES   NO

4. Did you often or very often feel that:

   No one in your family loved you or thought you were important or special **OR** your family didn't look out for each other, feel close to each other, or support each other?   YES   NO

5. Did you often or very often feel that:

   You didn't have enough to eat, had to wear dirty clothes, and had no one to protect you **OR** your parents were too drunk or high to take care of you or take you to the doctor if you needed it?   YES   NO

6. Was your mother or stepmother or father or stepfather:

   Often or very often pushed, grabbed, slapped, or had something thrown at her/him **OR** sometimes, often, or very often kicked, bitten, hit with a fist, or hit with something hard **OR** *ever* repeatedly hit for at least a few minutes or threatened with a knife or gun?   YES   NO

Adverse Childhood Experiences (ACEs) (*Continued*)

7. Were your parents ever separated or divorced?   YES NO

8. Did you live with anyone who was a problem-drinker   YES NO
   or alcoholic or who used street drugs or prescription
   drugs not as prescribed?

9. Was a household member depressed or mentally ill or   YES NO
   did a household member attempt suicide?

10. Did a household member go to prison?   YES NO

Protective and Compensatory Experiences (PACEs)

When you were growing up, prior to your 18th birthday:

1. Did you have someone who loved you unconditionally   YES NO
   (you did not doubt that they cared about you)?

2. Did you have at least one best friend (someone you   YES NO
   could trust, had fun with)?

3. Did you do anything regularly to help others (e.g.,   YES NO
   volunteer at a hospital, nursing home, faith-based)
   or do special projects in the community to help
   others (e.g., food drives, Habitat for Humanity)?

4. Were you regularly involved in organized sports   YES NO
   groups (e.g., soccer, basketball, track) or other
   physical activity (e.g., competitive cheer, gymnastics,
   dance, marching band)?

5. Were you an active member of at least one civic   YES NO
   group or a nonsport social group such as scouts,
   faith-based, or youth group?

(continues)

Protective and Compensatory Experiences (PACEs) **(Continued)**		
6. Did you have an engaging hobby—an artistic or intellectual pastime either alone or in a group (e.g., chess club, debate team, musical instrument or vocal group, theater, spelling bee, or did you read a lot)?	YES	NO
7. Was there an adult (not your parent) you trusted and could count on when you needed help or advice (e.g., coach, teacher, minister, neighbor, relative)?	YES	NO
8. Was your home typically clean AND safe with enough food to eat?	YES	NO
9. Overall, did your schools provide the resources and academic experiences you needed to learn?	YES	NO
10. In your home, were there rules that were clear and fairly administered?	YES	NO

RESOURCES

Burke-Harris, N. (2018). *The deepest well*. Houghton Mifflin Harcourt.

Hays-Grudo, J., & Morris, A. S. (n.d.). *We are the sum of our experiences: ACEs and PACEs*. https://www.acesandpaces.com

Hays-Grudo, J., & Morris, A. S. (2020). *Adverse and protective childhood experiences: A developmental perspective*. American Psychological Association. https://doi.org/10.1037/0000177-000

Schiraldi, G. R. (2021). *The adverse childhood experiences recovery workbook: Heal the hidden wounds from childhood affecting your adult mental and physical health*. New Harbinger Publications.

van der Kolk, B. (2014). *The body keeps the score: Brain, mind, and body in the healing of trauma*. Viking.

The following are some mental health resources in case you want to reach out after reading this chapter to get help concerning your own past trauma or history of ACEs. We encourage you to talk with someone if you have never shared your ACEs story before or if you feel you are in crisis for any reason.

- Access https://www.apa.org/topics/psychotherapy for the American Psychological Association's Psychologist Locator and other mental health resources.
- Dial 988 to access the U.S. Nationwide Suicide & Crisis Lifeline, available 24 hours.
- Text HELLO to 741741 for the Crisis Text Line.
- Access https://www.psychologytoday.com/us/therapists to find a licensed psychologist by zip code or city.
- Dial 1-800-662-HELP (4357), the U.S. Substance Abuse and Mental Health Services Administration's National Helpline, a treatment referral center staffed 24 hours a day for individuals and family members facing mental and/or substance use disorders.

CHAPTER 3

BABIES AND TODDLERS: BALANCING SAFETY AND EXPLORATION

The office manager took Jennifer's insurance information and ushered her into an exam room to wait for the doctor. She looked around the brightly decorated room and imagined how her life would change when the baby arrived. The door opened, and in walked a smiling Dr. Rey Calderón, the pediatrician who would care for her children for the next 20 years. This was the get-acquainted visit so they would be prepared if any issues arose during delivery. They talked about expectations and bringing the baby home, and then he asked her, "Will you have grandmas to help out when the baby comes?" Jennifer nodded yes. He followed up, "Whose mother?" Jennifer admitted what she usually managed not to think much about: "My mother-in-law is coming. My mother died when I was 14." Without breaking eye contact or missing a beat, Dr. Calderón said, "Oh, she will be there for you."

When a baby comes into the world, they are born into a family with a unique history, culture, neighborhood, and home. What Dr. Calderón recognized was that our childhoods affect how we interpret, react, and respond to our babies and children. In this chapter, we invite you to think about your childhood and how it influences how you feel about being a parent. If you are about to welcome or have recently welcomed a baby into your life, we extend our congratulations and well wishes. And we offer lots of practical advice that we think will be helpful as you begin your parenting journey.

MILE MARKERS

Having a new baby is one of the greatest challenges in life. You think pregnancy is hard, but then you realize that life was actually easier before the baby was born. During pregnancy, the baby is cared for in the womb, but after its birth, the baby needs to be fed and changed every few hours and held and rocked to sleep, and your own sleep comes in fits and starts. All of this is normal but trying for new and even experienced parents. And this is assuming that everything has gone according to plan and there are no medical problems (for more on this topic, see the Practical Tip 3.2: Medical Problems During Infancy later in this chapter). Amanda remembers the long ride in the wheelchair as she was leaving the hospital with her newborn son, Caleb, in her arms. He cried the entire trip from her room, through the corridors of the hospital, and down to the parking garage, for what seemed like forever. She felt stressed and helpless. She could not calm him, and she was supposed to be a parenting expert! Suddenly, she realized how much she had to learn about parenting this unique little person.

Despite their many challenges, the first 3 years of life are a special time for both babies and parents. It can be helpful for parents to understand development at each age and stage during this time. Using our road map analogy, knowing these "mile markers," or developmental milestones, can help you be prepared for the journey ahead. Understanding what to expect at different ages will also help you know how to tell if your child is on track or if interventions are needed. In Tables 3.1 and 3.2, we list a number of developmental milestones that are typical from birth to age 3 (Berk, 2015). Please note that there is a wide age range for each stage and that children vary a great deal in terms of when they reach different milestones. There is no need to worry unless children are out of the typical range. The Centers for Disease Control and Prevention provides detailed information on developmental milestones and when to talk to your pediatrician or seek other help at different ages (see Resources). Note that babies who grow up in a home with more than one language may be delayed on some of the language milestones, but they will catch up later—and then they have two or more languages they can speak and understand!

Babies

The first 3 months of a baby's life have been called the fourth trimester for good reason. It takes a while for babies to adjust to living outside their mothers' bodies, where all their needs were met automatically. Before they were born, no one cared (much) if they were awake at night and slept all day, and they had a continuous food delivery system. Now they must figure out how to sleep when the adult people sleep and how to let them know when they are hungry, are in pain or uncomfortable, or just need some cuddles. This is a challenging time for parents because it may seem like there is little reward for all the hard work of feeding, bathing, and diapering, especially when operating on little sleep and when mom's hormones are not yet stabilized after pregnancy.

Gradually, parents and babies begin to figure out each other's "language," like partners learning to dance together. Parents learn what babies' different cries mean and how to comfort them, and babies slowly become familiar with their surroundings. When the first smile comes around 6 to 8 weeks, it is thrilling and makes all the difference in the world. (See Table 3.1 for early milestones.)

Experts agree that moms should try to breastfeed their babies for many reasons. It is free, and breast milk provides increased

TABLE 3.1. Developmental Milestones in Infancy

Age	Physical	Language	Thinking and learning	Social and emotional
Birth to 6 months	• Has day and nighttime sleep patterns • Holds head up • Rolls over • Grasps objects	• Coos • Babbles at end of this age range • Looks at objects and activities labeled by others	• Imitates facial expressions • Repeats behaviors to get results	• Socially smiles and laughs • Knows positive versus negative emotions • Regulates emotions by self-soothing (e.g., sucking) and looking away • Matches feeling tone of caregivers
7 to 12 months	• Sits alone • Crawls • Walks	• Increases babbling • Takes turns in games (e.g., peekaboo) • Points to things • Understands some words • Says first word around 1 year	• Finds a hidden object • Understands simple directions	• Increases smiling and laughing • Exhibits stranger and separation anxiety • Explores environment • Has a preference for a caregiver • Can look to and interpret others' feelings

immunity and all the nutrients infants need. However, breastfeeding can be challenging for many mothers. You may struggle in the early days of breastfeeding. It sometimes takes longer than you expect for it to become natural and not painful, and caregivers can benefit by reaching out to organizations such as La Leche League and other local support groups for new parents (see Resources).

The first year of life is an amazing time for change, with babies starting to explore by crawling (most, but not all, babies crawl) and eventually walking, saying their first words, exploring objects, and feeding themselves. Despite the exhaustion and sleep deprivation most parents experience, it can be helpful to cherish each moment and remind yourself to enjoy these early days and nights. Amanda remembers rocking Caleb when he was tiny and thinking he would only be this size and this way at this one moment. Babies change so fast, and all too soon the newborn diapers are too small, and moms are putting away the 0- to 3-month clothes. You may want to take note of these changes by keeping a calendar or journal. This can be difficult when you have little time for yourself, but you will enjoy looking back on the notes you make, and children love to hear stories about what they did and were like when they were babies.

Zooming In 3.1: Baby Brain Development

Babies are born with more than 100 billion neurons. Their brains are about a quarter of the size of an adult brain. In the first year of life, the brain doubles in size and is almost full size by age 5. Although the size of the brain is comparable to an adult's, the architecture of the brain is constantly changing, with connections between neurons forming at a rapid pace during the first few years of life. What scientists have learned over the past few decades is that brain connections are driven by daily experiences and interactions. As humans, we are "wired to connect." This means that

(continues)

> ## Zooming In 3.1: Baby Brain Development (*Continued*)
>
> physical and emotional connections between babies and parents affect the "wiring" of the brain. Human interactions, not screens or fancy toys, are the building blocks of brain development. When babies feel safe and their world is predictable, the brain is primed for learning and language development. Scientists have found this in numerous studies comparing brain development among babies raised in nurturing, safe environments with babies living in impoverished, neglectful environments. Parents' daily interactions prime children for adapting to the world in which they live. This underscores the importance of positive interactions and the need to protect children from exposure to conflict, maltreatment, and neglect.

Toddlers

When babies start walking, usually around a year, things really change! Toddlerhood is often called "the terrible twos" for good reason. Toddlers want what they want and when they want it; they want to do things on their own and say "no" a lot. Toddlers don't yet have the language to fully communicate their needs, and this can be frustrating for all. Amanda's little sister had a t-shirt when she was a toddler that said, "Don't Bug Me I Bite." We don't want our toddlers to bite, but we do want them to become more independent and confident. One way to help them explore and be more independent is by childproofing some rooms in your home by covering electrical outlets, gating off stairs, and keeping out of reach anything that shouldn't be put in babies' mouths or swallowed. (For a checklist, see the Resource section. See Table 3.2 for developmental milestones for this age.)

It is also good for babies and toddlers to play outdoors where there are safe spaces for them to explore and burn off energy. You may find Dr. Penelope Leach's (2010) advice helpful when your

TABLE 3.2. Developmental Milestones in Toddlerhood

	Physical	Language	Thinking and learning	Social and emotional
1 to 2 years	• Walks in a more coordinated way • Picks up small objects • Feeds self • Jumps, walks on tiptoes, and climbs (19–24 months)	• Understands 50 words (13 months) • Produces 50 words (18 months) • Produces 200 words (19–24 months) • Combines 2 words (19–24 months)	• Repeats behaviors to learn • Memory for people, things, and events improves • Sorts objects into categories • Engages in make-believe play • Can follow simple directions • Uses own name and personal pronouns (19–24 months)	• Plays with others • Realizes others have different emotions • Looks to others to understand events and emotions • Shows empathy (e.g., may offer someone their blanket) • Talks about feelings (19–24 months) • Has less separation anxiety (19–24 months) • Can wait a short time for things (19–24 months)
2 to 3 years	• Hops, jumps, throws • Takes off and put on simple clothes • Uses a spoon • Scribbles	• Knows 200 words • Learns about five words a day • Speaks in simple sentences • Can have a simple conversation	• Increases pretend play • Takes the perspective of others in simple face-to-face interactions • Begins to count	• Understands basic emotions • Begins to exhibit self-concept and self-esteem • Evaluates own and others' actions (e.g., nice, mean) • May use aggression to get what they want

children are this age (see Resources). Dr. Leach is a British developmental psychologist who advises that parents of crawlers and toddlers be relaxed about letting their children explore their surroundings. We agree with her that toddlers should have dirty knees at bath time because that means they have been exploring and learning about their world!

One of the big accomplishments for our independent toddlers is learning how to control their bodies, transitioning from diapers to using the toilet. Some children may be ready as early as 18 to 24 months, but most toilet training occurs between 2 and 3 years of age. There are many helpful tools and strategies to help with potty training, and we won't go into great detail in this book except to assure parents that all typically developing children will learn to use the toilet. It is common for toddlers to go back and forth between diapers and the potty and relapse during times of transition (new sibling, starting preschool). Waiting until your child shows interest and is "potty ready" and being patient are two keys to success. You may find it helpful to check out the books in the Resources section at the end of Chapter 4. There are books, videos, and websites that provide parents with good information and ways to introduce the process in a positive way. It is helpful to have a child-size potty chair with a bowl that can be emptied or a potty seat that fits on the toilet so children can get on and off the toilet easily and safely. We suggest not worrying too much about boys standing up to urinate until they get a little older.

Be sure and talk with any childcare providers you may have before you start the process. Some childcare facilities have set routines and practices that they follow with all children. You will want to make sure these are practices that you understand, agree with, and can follow at home so that children don't get confused about what is expected of them in different settings. Likewise, if grandparents or others share childcare responsibilities, try to make sure everyone is using the same language and routines.

Use whatever rewards you and your child find helpful—praise and high fives or stickers and special treats—and be patient. The main guideline for toilet training is to take your cues from the child—don't introduce it until they indicate they are ready, and be prepared to stop and try again later if they struggle or lose interest in it.

Toddlerhood is also an incredible time of cognitive growth, when children learn hundreds of words a week, begin speaking in sentences, and master new thinking skills. Amanda remembers Caleb saying, "I do it," when she brushed his teeth and when he batting away the spoon so he could feed himself. This need for independence is often difficult for parents and can even lead to temper tantrums and "meltdowns." For example, when Jennifer's daughter Amy was almost 2, she knew what she wanted but wasn't yet verbal enough to communicate it. One night on vacation, the family went to dinner at a nice restaurant. The server took their order, but the food did not come right away. Suddenly they heard a "roar" come out of Amy, and before they could react, Amy had swiped her little arm across the table, sending silverware flying. Jennifer will never forget the look of awe on Amy's older brother's face, who was clearly thinking, "I didn't know we could do that!" Indeed, Zack was calm and easy-going and hadn't given his parents the opportunity to deal with tantrums. Amy was made of different stuff. Her brief but intense tantrums were the early indicators of the passion for fairness and social justice she would later display as an adolescent and young woman. Sometimes parents survive by reminding themselves that 2-year-olds haven't yet had time to learn how to channel all that emotion, energy, and curiosity, but they will with our love and support.

This is precisely why balanced parenting focuses on finding ways to allow both children's freedom to explore and learn with parents' direction and control, which is not always an easy task. Luckily, Amanda was patient with Caleb's teeth brushing, and Jennifer had snacks and books in her bag for Amy the next time they went to a restaurant. As a parent, you will make mistakes, and that is okay! Trust us, we made a lot and still do. What is important is to acknowledge your mistakes, think about what you learned, and move on. In some ways, parenting does get easier, but there are always new challenges as children grow and change. Often, when you think you have it figured out, a child brings a new challenge, or a sibling is born with a new set of characteristics, and the same parenting strategies just don't work.

BALANCING ACTS WITH BABIES AND TODDLERS

Driving on snowy roads or in a thunderstorm, parents can feel some assurance when they are in an all-wheel drive car. In an all-wheel drive vehicle, the power is distributed differentially to the wheels depending on where the car needs traction. This concept of shifting power according to the terrain is similar to the idea of balanced parenting, as we discussed in Chapter 1. Parenting should differ according to the child's developmental stage, the needs of the child, and even the situation. One of the best ways to manage the challenges of infancy and toddlerhood is through our balanced parenting approach. Balanced parenting helps both children and parents be more resilient and handle the challenges that arise at this stage of development. Table 3.3 lists the developmental challenges, balancing acts, and resilient child outcomes that result from a balanced parenting approach during the first 3 years of life. Balanced parenting provides a positive way to deal with the push and pull of children's need for independence and parents' need for control while maintaining warmth and nurturance as the foundation of the parent–child relationship.

TABLE 3.3. Balanced Parenting During Infancy and Toddlerhood

Stage and age	Developmental challenges	Balanced parenting	Resilient child outcomes
Infant (birth–1)	• Attachment versus separation	• Responsiveness versus self-care	• Trust (I am loved)
Toddler (1–2)	• Agency versus helplessness	• Safety versus exploration	• Courage (I can come and go)

Balanced Parenting in Infancy: Responsiveness and Self-Care

In the first year of life, parents must balance responding to babies with caring for themselves. This can be particularly hard for single parents and working moms and dads. Sleep deprivation and hormonal changes can lead to mood changes, ranging from mild cases of the "baby blues" to more serious episodes of postpartum depression. These risks to caregivers and babies are common, and family members and friends need to watch for symptoms such as feelings of sadness all the time, lack of joy in things that are usually happy, and changes in eating (lack of appetite or overeating). There may be days in those first few months when even taking a shower is impossible unless you have someone else to care for the baby for a while during the day or evening. Having grandparents, friends, or other relatives to help with the baby in these first few months can make a big difference. Parents should not feel guilty about asking for help, especially in the first few months after the baby is born. In fact, the first 3 months are particularly trying for most families and babies. It does get easier with time.

The challenge during this time, then, is responding consistently to babies' needs and still caring for oneself. It is important to soothe babies when they cry. Physical contact and comfort are almost always soothing to a baby. Sometimes babies are overstimulated and need quiet and calm. Experts agree that newborn babies cannot be "spoiled" by holding them, and meeting babies' needs is an essential parenting task. However, parents can neglect their own needs at the expense of the child in the long run. Thousands of studies show the negative impact of maternal depression and parental psycho-pathology on children's developmental outcomes. So, we must care for ourselves, or we won't be able to care for our babies.

It is sometimes difficult to know what newborns and young babies need. Even though parents want to be responsive, it takes time to learn how to read a baby's signals. There are clues that can help. Are they hungry (when did they last eat?), tired (when did they last sleep?), or overstimulated (are there too many sounds and toys?)? By observing babies' responses and setting up regular routines, you will learn the best ways to respond in the moment. For example, Jennifer learned within a few weeks that after a middle-of-the-night feeding, her son needed to be changed, swaddled, and put back in the crib to go back to sleep. When she rocked him afterward, he would fuss. A few years later, his little sister let her know that she needed some-thing different. She would let out a howl if put back in the crib after feeding and changing, but she slipped easily back into sleep after a good cuddle in the rocking chair.

When babies have their needs met consistently, they learn how to soothe themselves and trust others. Of course, they still experience distress, but they learn ways to calm down and accept comfort from a caregiver. Early on, this is done through simple strategies and reflexes such as sucking and looking away. When they're a little older, babies

Practical Tip 3.1: They Won't Stop Crying!

It is normal for babies to cry as much as 5 hours a day. This can start when babies are as young as 2 weeks and typically peaks when babies are around 6 to 8 weeks. Crying usually lessens around 3 to 5 months. The first few months can be difficult for parents because there is often little that parents can do to soothe a baby. Some things parents can do are:

- **swaddle:** This makes babies feel safe and helps them to settle. Wrapping their arms in a blanket also prevents them from accidentally upsetting themselves with uncontrolled arm movements.
- **watch the clock:** Keep a record of when and how long crying episodes occur. Often, crying seems a lot longer than it actually is, and parents can learn what to expect.
- **trade off:** Take turns with another parent or caregiver to give each other a break when possible.
- **walk or go outside:** Babies are soothed by gentle movement and a change of scenery. When you can manage it, long walks after dinner are great for everyone.
- **avoid overstimulation:** When a baby starts to fuss, they often need a break, and it may be time for a nap. Sometimes, if parents wait too long, babies get overly tired and cannot settle down.
- **put baby in the crib:** If you know your baby is clean and not hungry, it is okay to put the baby down, maybe with soft music. Video monitors make this easier—you can watch babies settle and be sure they are safe. Sometimes babies will fall asleep after a good cry, but be sure the crib is empty of all toys and blankets and that the room is quiet and not overly bright. And caregivers should **never shake a baby**. It only takes a few seconds for irreparable brain damage or even death to occur. It is always better to put a baby in a safe place and take a break when parents start to feel helpless or angry.

may reach up to a parent to be picked up or hug a blanket or stuffed toy for comfort. Babies explore their world through touch, taste, sight, and sound by putting things in their mouths, patting, touching, grabbing, holding, and moving through their world. They may drop things over and over onto the floor from their high chair. This can be frustrating for mom or dad, but this is how they learn. After all, we aren't born knowing about gravity! Babies also learn by interacting with others. Interactions with parents provide the foundation for how children understand the world and form future relationships.

The developmental challenge for babies during this time is *attachment versus separation*. Attachment is one of the most important concepts in psychology and parenting science and is key to balanced parenting during this stage. Attachment starts early in life and sets the foundation for later social relationships. When parents are responsive and consistent, children develop a secure attachment to caregivers. Secure attachment enables them to explore their world and come back to a parent when they are afraid or hurt, feeling safe and secure because their needs are met. Secure attachment develops because parents respond to babies' needs, soothe them when they cry, feed them when they are hungry, change their diapers when needed, and provide a consistent source of comfort. In contrast, insecure attachments occur when the infant's needs are met inconsistently or not at all. These babies learn that they cannot rely on their caregivers for consistent help and often send mixed signals to caregivers, sometimes resulting in learned helplessness where children stop crying to get their parents' attention or stop going to caregivers when they need them. Insecurely attached children often struggle with relationships throughout life, having difficulty making friends, connecting with teachers and other authority figures, and maintaining romantic relationships. They have trouble trusting others.

Experts agree that a baby's attachment is the foundation for healthy development and relationships across a lifetime. This first attachment leads to an ability to trust or mistrust others and makes it easier to connect with others in the future and to love and be loved. Please note that when we talk about attachment in this book, we are referring to developmental research and theory on attachment, not *attachment parenting*, which has been popularized in the press and advocates for co-sleeping and the near constant presence of a parent, which may not work for all families.

Zooming In 3.2: Working Models of Attachment and the Strange Situation

Scientists started theorizing about attachment during World War II when many children in London were sent to the country to be safe from the daily bombing known as the blitzkrieg. John Bowlby, a child psychiatrist in London, observed the impact of this family separation on children's behavior and mental health and developed the working model of attachment (Bowlby, 2008). In this theory, children's beliefs about relationships are the result of their early relationships with their parents and the availability and quality of those relationships. Years later, developmental psychologist Mary Ainsworth created a system for measuring children's attachment to their parents (Ainsworth et al., 1978). Separation anxiety and stranger wariness are common stressors for young children; Ainsworth used these stressors to observe how children interacted with their caregivers. She developed the Strange Situation, a laboratory paradigm for toddlers where children encounter a structured series of interactions that involve a stranger, separation, and reunion with a caregiver, and a classification system based on children's reactions. *Securely attached* children are easily soothed by a caregiver, indicating consistent care and nurturance. *Insecurely attached* children are either avoidant or anxious. *Insecurely attached–avoidant* children soothe themselves on their own and tend to avoid the parent. These infants are believed to have parents who do not respond regularly to their children's bids for attention, resulting in

(continues)

Zooming In 3.2: Working Models of Attachment and the Strange Situation (*Continued*)

children who soothe themselves and may feel that they are not heard or important. *Insecurely attached–anxious children* act as if they want to be soothed but continue to show distress. *Anxious* infants are believed to have parents who are inconsistent: Sometimes they are responsive, and other times they are not, resulting in a lack of predictability and overall anxiety in children. Children with *disorganized attachment* respond to their caregiver in unusual ways (e.g., freezing, hiding), and this is often a sign of maltreatment.

Balanced Parenting in Toddlerhood: Safety and Exploration

The balancing act for parents of toddlers is keeping toddlers safe while also letting them explore. Between the ages of 1 and 3, children love to explore. As they become able to walk, climb, and run, they need opportunities to learn about the world safely. Toddlers need to go for walks and play outdoors, visit parks and libraries, and be around other children. In a way, toddlers are like little scientists who learn about the world by seeking out new experiences; testing how things feel, taste, and work; and using the information they gather to construct an understanding of the world. Toddlers are also beginning to learn the basics of self-control—how to wait for things, look but not touch, and follow simple instructions and routines. Ideally, toddlers feel safe to explore their environments and regularly check back in with caregivers.

The concept of the Circle of Security (Hoffman et al., 2006; see Figure 3.1) beautifully illustrates the idea of attachment and exploration during toddlerhood. Parents are the source of support, always bigger and stronger, the hands on the circle. Children venture out on the top of the circle to explore their world, and when they are

FIGURE 3.1. Circle of Security

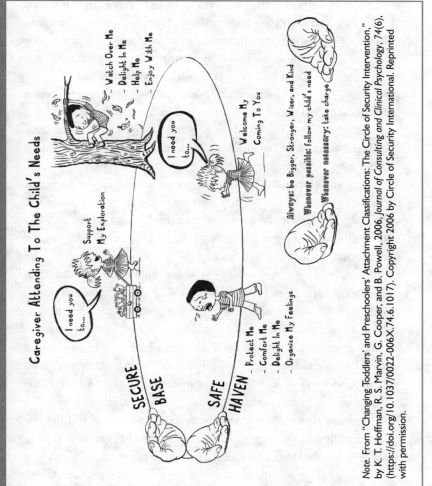

Note. From "Changing Toddlers' and Preschoolers' Attachment Classifications: The Circle of Security Intervention," by K. T. Hoffman, R. S. Marvin, G. Cooper, and B. Powell, 2006, *Journal of Consulting and Clinical Psychology, 74*(6), (https://doi.org/10.1037/0022-006X.74.6.1017). Copyright 2006 by Circle of Security International. Reprinted with permission.

scared or need a little help, they check back in and return to parents for comfort, as is illustrated on the bottom of the circle (Marvin et al., 2002). Importantly, along the way, children signal to parents their needs, and their parents' responses contribute to the formation of secure or insecure attachments. If children are comforted when in distress and if their exploration is supported, they become more securely attached. In contrast, if children are not consistently protected and comforted, secure attachments are less likely to develop. Examples of balanced parenting at this age include keeping an eye out while allowing children to venture away and being available but not hovering or showing concern unless they venture into harm's way.

The developmental challenge parents are helping their toddlers face is *agency versus helplessness*. Agency occurs when children feel that they can control their behavior, have choices, and have some influence on what happens to them. Later, they will begin to feel responsible for their actions and the consequences. In babies and toddlers, agency begins to develop when their actions lead to their needs being met. They begin to realize that what they do has some effect on their well-being. When they feel hungry and cry, they get picked up and fed. When they babble and wave their arms around, a familiar smiling face appears and makes babbling noises back to them. During toddlerhood, this is increasingly important as children become more active in their world by walking and talking. When toddlers are able to communicate their needs and are listened to, they develop this sense of agency. In contrast, when toddlers are ignored, yelled at, or responded to inconsistently, they may develop a sense of helplessness and feel that they do not matter or have any control over their world. Having a sense of agency allows children to feel safe and not be afraid to explore, try new things, and ask for help when they need it. The balancing act is helping toddlers keep that courageous, adventurous spirit while ensuring their safety from harm. Toddlers need courage to venture out and explore, and by creating places where they can safely explore, they develop a sense that they can make things happen, that they are important and not helpless. Just as babies and toddlers need courage to explore and learn, parents need the courage to explore how to respond to the individual needs of their baby and toddler. Both parents and babies need to feel safe and secure, trusting each other physically and mentally because this relationship will last a lifetime. Thus, the resilient outcome of balanced parenting during infancy and toddlerhood is trust and courage. This may be difficult for parents with a history of adverse childhood experiences (ACEs) or whose children have experienced adversity or trauma during their first 3 years.

PARENTING WHEN YOU HAVE ACEs: GHOSTS AND ANGELS IN THE NURSERY

In the story that opens this chapter, Dr. Calderon correctly assumed that Jennifer had good memories of her mother, ones that would be available to her as she became a mother. Sure enough, she found herself crooning lullabies and phrases as she rocked and comforted her newborn son—words and melodies that came from deep wells of memories from her childhood. Many parents are not so fortunate. When babies are born in adverse conditions—for example, when the parents are in open conflict, the mother is depressed, or the father drinks too much and is abusive—the memories children unconsciously store may be very different. When these children become parents, painful memories can hover in the background, unconsciously poisoning their feelings about being a parent and creating fear instead of joy. Therapists called infant mental health specialists, who specialize in helping parents who are having trouble caring for or feeling close to their babies because of traumatic childhoods, will often help parents identify and dismiss these *ghosts in the nursery*.

These intruders are the memories of things said and done that made the baby (now a parent) feel unwelcome, unloved, and unsafe in their homes, memories laid down before they had the language or logic to challenge them (Fraiberg et al., 2018). Like the Ghostbuster movies, these "ghosts" can be banished by bringing them into the open, into conscious memory, and confronting them as unhelpful and unwanted memories of the past. Infant mental health specialists also help parents who have had traumatic early childhoods to identify *angels in the nursery*, beneficial memories of being with someone who made them feel loved and safe, memories they can draw on as they become parents (Lieberman et al., 2005).

At the end of this chapter, we invite you to trace the patterns of ACEs and PACEs (protective and compensatory experiences) in your own family trees. This activity may surprise you. Recognizing these patterns is an important first step in changing them as you help your children chart a course for their lives that builds on the resilience of our ancestors without carrying forward the legacy of adversity.

Parenting with a history of ACEs is similar to parenting without ACEs—it just requires a bit more intentional thought. Most people parent the way their parents did it without thinking much about it. How many times have you heard, "Well, if it was good enough for me, it's good enough for my kids." That's the easy way to parent—easy in the short term because it requires so little thought. But parents who want to avoid the kinds of mistakes their parents made must decide how they want to respond when their children need attention, cry, get into mischief, or almost get hurt. Rather than automatically giving them a swat or ignoring their cries "so they learn who is boss," parents who want to break the cycle of ACEs in their families look for and learn new ways to respond. They talk about their intentions with their partners, friends, and families. Sometimes they get pushback from family members who cling to the old ways. Sometimes they make mistakes, but they keep trying. And they get help when they need it.

Jennifer was once flying home to Houston on a crowded flight when the man seated next to her mentioned that he was going home to a town just outside of Houston. Jennifer shared that her best friend worked at the county child and family services agency in that town. His face lit up in a smile, and he said that agency had "saved his family." He went on to tell her that he had been abused as a child by his father and swore that he would be different. But when his son turned 2 and talked back to him, he felt a strong urge to hit him. That automatic reaction shocked and scared him, so he made an appointment with a therapist at the local child and family services agency. He told her how grateful he was to the therapist there for teaching him how to replace the parenting behaviors he had experienced as a child with more effective, less harsh, and more loving responses. He proudly told Jennifer that he and his 16-year-old son now have a great relationship, and he had never once hit or hurt him.

Parents may also want to seek the help of professionals when their early reactions to an infant's dependency on them create resentment, anger, or fear. Although taking care of an infant is demanding, most parents find it rewarding to find themselves the center of their baby's world. But when a parent was abused or neglected as a child, they may react differently. One way that we can understand how the sound of a crying baby can either trigger feelings of love and care or feelings of panic and anger is to do the following thought exercise:

> Picture a beautiful beach with white sand, the waves softly lapping the shore and palm trees gently swaying as you imagine yourself walking along the shoreline. Complete the image with relaxing background music and enjoy for a few moments the feeling of peace and calm of the scene. . . . Now imagine the same scene, but the music changes suddenly to the ominous background music from the *Jaws* movies. You hear the deep

rumbling of bass notes signaling DANGER—there are sharks in the water! DUH-DUH, DUH-DUH, the music gets louder and faster.

Without seeing a single shark fin, the music alone is enough to shatter the calm, create fear, and make you want to run from the beach. This exercise, called "the shark music exercise" by our friends who developed the Circle of Security, illustrates how quickly and powerfully the background thoughts and memories from our childhoods can change our feelings from peace and joy to fear and anxiety. If you find yourself having angry or anxious reactions to your baby's cries or demands to be held, this is a good indicator that there are some harmful childhood experiences that need to be banished, some ghostbusting work to do. Getting professional help can be a life-changing experience for both parents and their children, and we encourage you to ask your pediatrician or other health care provider for a referral.

PARENTING STRATEGIES FOR BUILDING RESILIENCE

In this section, we offer general parenting strategies that benefit babies and toddlers in all families.

Routines

Babies and toddlers need order and routine, such as playtime, meal-time, bath time, and bedtime. Routines give children a sense of famil-iarity and predictability that makes them feel safe. It gives children a kind of script, so they know what to expect throughout the day. Schedules can differ on weekdays versus weekends, or as Amanda's kids would say, "school days or family days." It can be helpful to create a visual schedule using pictures or icons to post somewhere chil-dren can see. The schedule should be flexible but follow a predictable order most days. Routines also help children shift their attention and actions. For example, bedtime routines help children make the transition between being awake and falling asleep. And disrupting routines can be especially challenging. For example, sometimes going to the grocery store during bedtime hours is unavoidable, but you may notice how much more difficult it is to get a toddler to fall asleep afterward. Having a bedtime routine that starts with a bath and ends with a picture book or story helps children settle. As they get older, having a story or quiet conversation and a cuddle at bedtime gives toddlers something to look forward to at the end of their day. They learn what to expect, and it prevents arguments or tantrums. Babies and young children need much more sleep than adults. The American Academy of Pediatrics recommends that 4- to 12-month-olds get 12 to 16 hours (including naps) and toddlers 1 to 2 years old get 11 to 14 hours (including naps). Getting babies and toddlers to bed early also gives parents a much-needed break. After babies are in bed is a great time for taking care of yourself—talking with your partner, reading a book, texting a friend, or catching up on your own sleep.

Playtime

It is impossible to overemphasize the importance of play for young children. It has been said that children's play is their work because play is how they learn. With babies, play may be a game of peek-a-boo, stacking blocks, or playing with stuffed animals. With toddlers, it is good to let them choose the activity and take the lead. Letting toddlers direct the activity helps children develop emerging language and imagination skills and helps them learn to work out problems or difficulties. When parents are too directive during playtime, play isn't really play but just another time they have to figure out how to follow directions! Babies and toddlers love imitation, so if a child picks up a block and stacks it, do the same. If a child drinks from a teacup, then follow along and pretend to drink. Toddlers also love messy play because it is sensory and helps them learn about objects and materials. Examples include making shapes with shaving cream on the bathtub wall, building sandcastles in a sandbox or on the beach, pouring water from one container to another, or finger painting. Toddlers are developing small and large muscle groups, and this growth is enhanced through hands-on activities, both indoor and outdoor. Outdoor activities give toddlers a chance to develop large muscle groups and learn about the bigger world. Singing silly songs and making up stories are also great ways to play with toddlers when you're stuck in the car in traffic, waiting in line, or indoors on a rainy day.

Talking, Reading, Singing

There is abundant evidence that talking, reading, and singing to children every day helps them develop the language skills they need to communicate. Language begins to develop long before babies even say their first words, typically around 12 months. By about 9 months, babies understand words and can learn basic hand signs, such as milk, eat, light, night night, and please. There are many excellent websites and books on baby signs (see Resources), and signing can help babies communicate earlier than speech, easing some of their frustration. Another way to help babies communicate is to talk with them about what is going on in the world around them. Talk with them as you change their diaper, prepare dinner, shop for groceries, or go for a walk. Describe what you see, how something feels, tastes, or smells, using simple words and language. Name colors, objects, and sounds. Reading stories or picture books is also a great way to help children learn language and can help children transition from active time to rest time. This can start with simple board or cloth books and then advance to more complex picture books. Rather than just reading, talk about what is going on in a story and about the pictures in the book. Read at times other than nap or bedtime. Toddlers love it when parents use funny voices for different characters, and they love choosing which books to read, even if it is the same book every night. Jennifer's son, as a toddler, often asked her to tell a story "out of her mouth" rather than out of a book, so be prepared to make up stories! This can be a good way to help children remember and talk about the activities that happened during the day or special family events or highlight the things they've learned to do.

Limiting Screen Time

Screens should be avoided as much as possible during infancy and toddlerhood. This is one of the hardest strategies for parents to implement in today's world, where we are surrounded by handheld, desktop, and big screens that we depend on for information, work, and entertainment. The American Academy of Pediatrics recommends no screen time before children are 18 months old and no more than an hour a day between 18 months and 5 years. However, they also recommend that if you allow a 2-year-old to watch a program, you watch with them so that you can explain and talk about what they are seeing. During this age, your child needs to be exploring and understanding the real world rather than being distracted by movement and sounds from two-dimensional representations of the world. Ideally, parents should limit screens during the first 2 years to social interactions, such as FaceTime with grandparents or other friends and family members. This also requires parents to put away their smartphones as much as possible when with their kids.

Discipline: Creating Safe Spaces

Many parents start to worry about discipline during toddlerhood. When children start crawling, walking, and getting into things, it's natural for parents to worry. The best thing parents can do to prevent children from making messes, breaking things, or getting hurt is to set up a safe environment for exploration. Have a safe place for children to play in each room—a cabinet in the kitchen with spoons and plastic bowls, a box of blocks and toys in the living room, books and stuffed animals in the bedroom. When children begin to walk, teach them to follow simple rules, such as "look with your eyes, not with your hands" or "use one finger" when touching something fragile. Jennifer taught her toddlers that all glass items were "delicate" and only to be looked at and pointed to but not touched. Jennifer's family once went to dinner at a friend's house whose living room had an entire wall of glass shelves displaying fragile figurines and other obviously valuable objects. As they walked into the room, and before Jennifer could even say a word, her 2-year-old daughter began pointing to each object, saying "delicate, delicate, delicate" until each one was labeled. Crisis avoided! With some active toddlers, breakables need to be put safely out of reach until they are older. And with all babies, once they can move around on their own, it is essential to make the home safe by putting in plug covers, putting gates on stairs, and making sure they can't get into household cleaners and choke on small objects. One rule of thumb is that if an object fits inside a cardboard toilet paper roll holder, it is too small for children and is a choking hazard. Many products can help "babyproof" your home by preventing little ones from opening drawers and cabinets where unsafe products and utensils are stored. For a complete list for making your home safe for children, see the resources at the end of this chapter.

Discipline: Distraction

Distraction is a parent's best friend during this age. Because the world is so new to them, toddlers are easily distracted. When you want to stop them from grabbing a toy from another child, you can usually avoid a meltdown by giving them a different object to play with. When you want to get them into the tub for a bath or into the car to go home, you can remind them about the bath toys in the tub waiting to be played with or sing a silly song that you only sing while driving in the car. Helping children communicate their needs, keeping them busy, and creating a safe place for exploration are all keys to creating a calm and peaceful environment that fosters healthy development and builds resilience.

When meltdowns or tantrums happen, and they will, experts agree that parents should not give in to or reinforce a tantrum by allowing a child to get their way. Be sure the child is safe, and give it a little time. Usually, children will calm down on their own when they realize the tantrum is not working. Parents can try ignoring the behavior, or they can speak in a calm voice to their child to help them settle down. If tantrums become more extreme (a child hits their head against the wall or holds their breath), it may indicate other problems, and professional help may be needed.

DEALING WITH UNEXPECTED CHALLENGES

In August of 2005, Amanda's home in New Orleans was flooded by Hurricane Katrina. Before the storm, she and her husband, Mike, evacuated to her parents' house in Houston with 3-month-old Mollie, 2-year-old Caleb, two cats, and a golden retriever. Even worse than losing their home was the fear of not knowing where they would live, if they would have jobs, and what to do next. They went into action mode, solving problems and making decisions, but the experience was numbing. Amanda remembers the sick feeling of returning to a moldy, smelly house littered with the ruined remnants from their pre-Katrina life. As she shoveled out their children's moldy stuffed animals and other debris, Amanda wondered how she could protect her children from the anguish she was experiencing and whether this trauma would damage them in some way.

In any traumatizing situation, parents wonder how to protect their children. It is hard to be present and loving when your head is spinning and you are in survival mode. During these times it is most important and most difficult to engage in balanced parenting. In the Hurricane Katrina situation, Amanda and her family were relatively fortunate. They had family and friends they could count on and had access to other resources. While they waited for the city to be livable again, they stayed with Amanda's parents, filing insurance claims and looking for a new place to live. They found a preschool program for Caleb and set up new routines. They didn't bring their children back to New Orleans until they had a new place to live and kept them from seeing the images of destruction on television. They explained to 2-year-old Caleb what happened in terms he could understand. They focused on rebuilding, not on the devastation and destruction. Still, he knew what had happened and would say things like, "Look, it's not all wet" when he got a new book or toy and "That yucky old Katrina" when he saw a flooded home or a destroyed building back in New Orleans. But he was able to cope with the disruptions because he was shielded as much as possible, both from his parents' feelings and from the actual devastation. Later, they made the difficult decision to leave New Orleans and relocate to Oklahoma. Although Mike and Amanda may never know all the ways Katrina affected them, they do know they did their best to weather the storm, literally and figuratively, and prevent any lasting trauma to their children and themselves.

As Amanda's Katrina story illustrates, parents have a great deal of control over how young children perceive and view the world. Disasters happen, whether earthquakes, hurricanes, wildfires, tornados, or other unforeseeable tragic events. When parents have support and resources to cope with such events, they can try to shield and filter how much of the emotional drama and physical hardship their children are exposed to. It is not always possible to fully protect children from adversity, nor are we advocating for children to be wrapped in cotton balls and completely sheltered from the real world. We are saying, however, that during situations that can provoke trauma and lasting damage, parents should prioritize protecting their children as much as they can while making sure that they themselves get the support and resources they need. Accepting assistance from friends and family is key to building resilience during such times. Also important is creating new routines that accommodate any changes the family is experiencing. New routines create a sense that there is a "new normal" and help both young children and parents feel safe.

Other potentially traumatic situations during infancy can result from complications during childbirth, premature delivery, congenital anomalies, birth defects, or other health problems requiring specialized medical care (see Practical Tip 3.2: Medical Problems During Infancy). When unexpected traumas arise during the first few years of a child's life, parents cope more easily when they follow a balanced parenting approach. Finding the right balance that allows you to take care of yourself while meeting baby's needs and having set up an environment that keeps children safe while giving them freedom to explore allows parents the energy and focus they need to navigate unexpected hardships. When parents haven't found that balance and every day is a struggle to take care of oneself or a battle over bath and bedtime, it is doubly difficult to cope with additional challenges.

In Chapter 2, we described how ACEs can affect the body, brain, and behavior for a lifetime. For parents who have a history of ACEs, now is the time to spend the effort to recognize the effects of ACEs and create more individual and family PACEs to become more resilient. Sometimes even babies and toddlers have already experienced trauma, as may be the case with adoption, health problems and medical procedures, or other circumstances beyond our control. In the next section, we provide some recommendations and practical tips for parenting children with a history of ACEs.

Practical Tip 3.2: Medical Problems During Infancy

Few parents expect it, but about 10% of all babies born in the United States require at least some care in the neonatal intensive care unit (NICU), and this number has almost doubled in the past 15 years. Prematurity is the top reason babies are admitted to the NICU, but full-term babies may also need care for respiratory conditions, infections, hypoglycemia (low levels of glucose in their blood), jaundice, heart problems, or other conditions. Some babies stay a few days, and some stay for months, but all parents experience stress when their baby needs special care and worry that the experience will cause some lasting trauma. Fear (Is she going to be okay?), anger (How could this happen?), guilt (Could I have prevented this?), loss (This wasn't what I was expecting), and helplessness (I don't know what to do to help her) are normal feelings parents have in these situations. The following strategies have helped parents cope with the stress of having a baby in the NICU (see Resources for more information):

- connecting with the doctor and nurses so you know who to contact for information
- taking care of yourself, balancing time with the baby with getting enough sleep and exercise to reduce stress, eating healthy foods
- accepting help from others—ask favors and accept offers of assistance from family and friends
- being prepared for the unexpected, for a roller coaster of emotions, and knowing that you're not alone, that millions of other parents and babies have survived and thrived after NICU admissions
- if the stay in the NICU will be more than a few days, making it feel like home by personalizing it with photos or other decorations
- being involved with the clinic staff—touching and holding the baby (called kangaroo care) has medical benefits. When the medical team allows, participate in feeding, changing diapers and other care, and pump breastmilk to feed the baby and maintain a supply.

Note. Data from Ludington-Hoe and Swinth (1996).

PARENTING CHILDREN WHO HAVE A HISTORY OF ACEs

Babies and toddlers who have undergone traumatic situations or conditions benefit when their parents or other caregivers practice a balanced parenting approach and regulate their own emotions (more on this in Chapter 4). Balancing the need for self-care with the needs of a fussy baby or dysregulated toddler may involve more than making time to have a soak in the tub or read a magazine. Babies who have experienced trauma often have difficulty falling asleep at bedtime or after they wake in the night, may not want to be held or may want to be held all the time, and may be difficult to soothe. Toddlers who have endured adverse situations may respond with intense feelings when told they can't have or do something, may be either clingy or aloof, or may be easily distracted and have difficulty transitioning from one activity to another. They may be delayed in their development of language or motor skills. In extreme cases, like when children have been severely neglected and in institutionalized care, some children may never fully recover (Zeanah et al., 2019). As with adults who are still struggling with the very real biological and behavioral effects of adversity, getting professional support can be life changing for children as well as their caregivers. Each child is different, and different strategies are likely to work better or worse with different children.

All children benefit from PACEs, but they are especially important for young children who have undergone traumatic events or situations. PACEs for babies and toddlers are outlined in the table in Chapter 2 and include the following:

- nurturing and responsive care from parents or other caregivers
- spending time with other caring adults
- playing one-on-one with a peer or sibling
- playing with small groups of similar age-mates
- seeing and learning about empathy and caring for others

- having routines for bedtime, bath time, playtime, and mealtime
- having a home that is uncluttered and is a safe place to play and eat healthy food
- having opportunities to learn through play and being talked to and read to
- having time to play outdoors or be involved in other physical play
- having access to materials, such as paper, coloring tools, finger-puppets, or dress-up clothes to pretend and play creatively

Without question, the most important PACE is consistent, nurturing care from the adult who spends the most time with the child. Usually, that is the mother or father. But young children also benefit from relationships with other adults such as grandparents or childcare providers. Building these relationships early is beneficial for the whole family; parents can get a break, and children can have other special people to rely on and love. At an early age, young children also benefit from being around other children, such as siblings and peers of a similar age. When children are young, interactions with peers involve what we call parallel play, and although it seems like children are playing more on their own and not interacting, they are observing each other and benefiting from learning how to coordinate play and even share with others. Babies and toddlers also need safe places to play and have basic needs met and opportunities to learn through playing with safe objects and being active and having routines.

Remember, the "work" of toddlers and young children is play, and creating a schedule with play time boosts their cognitive, language, and social development. Toys do not have to be expensive. In fact, the best toys for helping toddlers and young children develop are simple objects like blocks and basic art materials. Taking advantage of local parks and libraries are free resources that most families have access to. Joining playgroups with other parents and children can be a great way for parents to enjoy friends and support while their children are playing together, especially if this is part of a regular routine. When parents need to work or need time for themselves, babies and toddlers benefit from quality care from another loved one or a quality preschool (discussed more in Chapter 4). It is important to be sure that childcare outside of the home meets the basic state standards, so look for childcare that meets national accreditation standards for quality care environments, if possible (see Resources).

If all this sounds overwhelming, it can be at times. But taking the time and energy to create PACEs will become easier as PACEs become part of your habits and routines. And those same PACEs will help you feel more in control of your time, your thoughts and emotions, and your life. Creating a home where traumatized children feel safe and calm allows their nervous systems to repair. Babies and toddlers are wired to connect and learn, and most will respond positively to responsive care, routines, and enriching environments, lessening the effects of ACEs.

KEY TAKEAWAYS

It is time to recap the main points of the chapter and think about your goals and plans for becoming a resilient parent and building resilience in your young child.

- Both negative (ghosts) and positive (angels) memories can take up residence in our children's nurseries, influencing our feelings about being a parent and our interactions with our babies and toddlers. The first step in breaking an intergenerational cycle of adversity is to recognize and reflect on family patterns of both adversity and protection and how they may be affecting our parenting.

- Take care of yourself. Get enough sleep and exercise, and eat well. Watch for signs of postpartum depression in the months after baby is born. Balancing time for yourself with caring for the baby will benefit both you and the baby. Accept and ask for help from others when needed.
- Set up routines. For young babies, it is worth the effort to try to maintain regular times for feeding, play, bath, and sleep. Toddlers benefit from having regular playtimes with other children (one-on-one and in small groups), parents, grandparents, and other caregivers; active play outdoors; and enjoyable bedtime routines. It is never too early to start reading to your baby and telling stories.
- Create a safe space for babies and toddlers to explore and play. Childproof your home before babies start crawling or walking. Spend time outdoors, first in the stroller on walks and later together at parks and in nature.
- Avoid harsh and intrusive parenting. Let your child take the lead in play and follow along, imitating and describing the activities you are doing together.
- Delight in your child. Keep a photo or journal record of all your baby's "firsts"—first bath, smile, laugh, rollover, word, and so forth. As challenging as it often is to welcome into the world and get to know a new little person, it is the beginning of an amazing adventure together.

ACTIVITY: YOU ARE HERE

We talked about the destination in Chapter 1—goals you are setting to create a home that builds resilience for you and your child. Take a minute to think about where you are now with balancing the competing demands of parenting your child and creating PACEs. Like a satellite navigating system on a smartphone, the following questions will allow you to mentally press the "you are here" icon and see where you are relative to where you want to go.

- What am I doing well as a parent? What do I enjoy most about parenting? What do I like most about my child?
- How are my parenting values affecting my interactions with my baby and toddler? Am I consistent in how and when I respond to my child?
- Where are you in terms of self-care versus responsiveness? Do you make time every day for your own needs—a shower, a walk, a chat with a friend, a healthy meal—or are you spending all your time hovering around the baby? Do you need to recalibrate or get more support?
- Where are you in terms of safety versus exploration? Have you childproofed all or part of your home so that your crawling baby or walking, climbing toddler can play without you having to constantly redirect or scold him? Take a few minutes to write down your ideas on where you are with this balancing act and anything you would like to do differently.
- What PACEs does your child already have? What PACEs would you like to add next? What PACEs do you have for yourself to keep your energy and mood stable during the demanding period of infancy and toddlerhood? What PACEs would you like to have? Take a few minutes to write on a calendar or a piece of paper the PACEs for yourself and your baby or toddler that you will add this week and decide how to do it. You can add a PACE or two each month as babies develop and your needs change.

ACTIVITY: ACEs AND PACEs GENOGRAMS

Families have a way of transmitting their history across generations. Identifying those patterns—both the positive and the negative ones—is helpful when we want to alter them. When medical genetic counselors look for genes in one's family that could cause problems for couples when they have children, they create a *genogram* that lists any genetic variations in one's ancestry. We use this format to identify patterns of ACEs and PACEs in our family histories that might influence our parenting with or without our knowing it, so we can create new patterns.

Begin in the box for yourself by listing the ACEs you had in your childhood. Next, list the PACEs you had from birth to 18. Then think back to the stories you have heard from your parents and grandparents. If they are open to the idea, ask them to tell you about their experiences, both adverse and protective. Notice if there are patterns or similarities across generations. Look at the differences or similarities between the history of your parents. Add boxes for stepparents or others who were involved in caring for you during your childhood.

Think about the strengths and positive qualities you would like to pass along to your children, and note the adversities you do not want to pass on. If you were writing a story about your family, what main themes would you highlight? How does it begin? How would you like it to end?

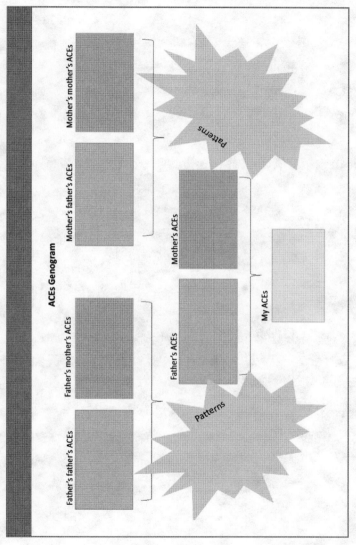

ACEs Genogram

Father's father's ACEs

Father's mother's ACEs

Mother's father's ACEs

Mother's mother's ACEs

Patterns

Patterns

Father's ACEs

Mother's ACEs

My ACEs

Notes:

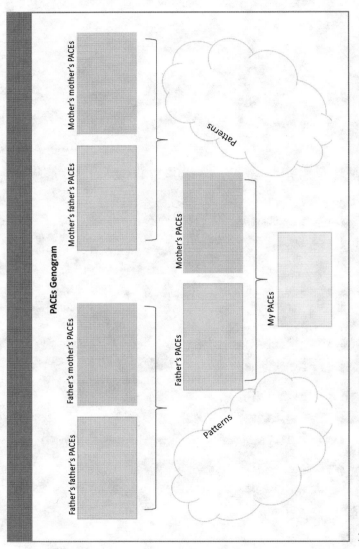

PACEs Genogram

| Father's father's PACEs | Father's mother's PACEs | Mother's father's PACEs | Mother's mother's PACEs |

Patterns

Father's PACEs | Mother's PACEs

Patterns

My PACEs

Notes:

RESOURCES

Breastfeeding Support

La Leche League International: +1-919-459-2167; +1-800-LALECHE (525-3243); https://llli.org

Office on Women's Health, U.S. Department of Health & Human Services: https://www.womenshealth.gov/breastfeeding

Developmental Milestones

Centers for Disease Control and Prevention: https://www.cdc.gov/ncbddd/actearly/milestones/index.html

U.S. National Library of Medicine: https://medlineplus.gov/ency/article/002002.htm

Special Challenges During Infancy

Infant crying: https://dontshake.org/purple-crying

NICU support for parents: https://www.marchofdimes.org/nicufamilysupport/index.aspx

Postpartum depression: https://www.nimh.nih.gov/health/publications/perinatal-depression

Resources for parents struggling to connect with or care for their baby or toddler (infant mental health): https://www.zerotothree.org/resources/for-families/

Childproofing Your Home

Childproofing checklists: https://www.childproofingexperts.com/childproofing-checklist.pdf

The U.S. Consumer Product Safety Commission guide for child safety devices: https://www.cpsc.gov/safety-education/safety-guides/kids-and-babies/childproofing-your-home-12-safety-devices-protect

99

General Parenting of Babies and Young Children

Brucks, B. (2016). *Potty training in 3 days: The step-by-step plan for a clean break from dirty diapers.* Althea Press.

Greenberg, G., & Hayden, J. (2004). *Be prepared: A practical handbook for new dads.* Simon & Schuster.

Hoffman, K., Cooper, G. G., & Powell, B. (2017). *Raising a secure child: How Circle of Security parenting can help you nurture your child's attachment, emotional resilience and freedom to explore.* Guilford Press.

Hogg, T., & Blau, M. (2001). *Secrets of the baby whisperer: How to calm, connect, and communicate with your baby.* Ballantine Books.

Karp, H. (2015). *The happiest baby on the block.* Bantam.

Leach, P. (2010). *Your baby and child: The classic childcare guide* (Rev. & updated). Knopf.

Popkin, M. H. (n.d.). Active parenting: First five years. https://activeparenting.com/product/first-five-years-of-parenting/

Resources for Teaching Preverbal Babies and Toddlers Sign Language

Acredolo, L., Goodwyn, S., & Abrams, D. (2009). *Baby signs: How to talk with your baby before your baby can talk* (3rd ed.). McGraw-Hill.

Kase, L. M., & Feld, G. B. (2020, January). Teaching baby sign language: A guide for new parents. *Parents.*

What to Look for When Deciding on a Childcare Program

https://www.naeyc.org/our-work/families/10-naeyc-program-standards

CHAPTER 4

EARLY CHILDHOOD: BALANCING CONTROL AND CHOICE

It was bath time at the Morris household. Five-year-old Caleb and 3-year-old Mollie came in from the backyard looking guilty. They had been playing together in the sandbox while Amanda cleaned up after dinner. The one sandbox rule (besides playing nice with each other) was never to put sand in each other's hair. Both children had thick hair that was difficult to wash sand out of. It didn't take long for Amanda to notice that Caleb's scalp was covered with a thick layer of sand and for Mollie to admit that she had dumped a bucket of sand on his head. Amanda took a few deep breaths before she said as calmly and firmly as she could, "Well, you know what this means—you will only get one book tonight instead of two—no bonus book." The second or "bonus" book was Mollie's reward for good behavior throughout the day. Mollie immediately began to argue: "But I NEED two books tonight; take away one TOMORROW. I will be good the WHOLE rest of the night. I will be good the WHOLE rest of the week. I'll NEVER put sand in Caleb's hair again." This went on for some time, and Amanda continued to say no, reminding Mollie that she knew the rules. Suddenly, Mollie stopped crying as an idea occurred to her. She quietly asked, "Can I have two half-books?" Amanda almost said no again automatically. But then she thought about it. Technically, it was still just one book.

She realized that her 3-year-old had just come up with a clever compromise that would allow her to follow the rules but also enjoy two different stories, at least parts of them. So that night, they read two half-books.

During early childhood, between the ages of 3 and 5, children develop distinct likes and dislikes. Their personalities become more defined, and you begin to glimpse the characteristics of the adults they will become. With the emergence of their wants and preferences also comes their desire to have what they want, when they want it, and how they want it. Like Mollie, they begin to use their developing language and logic skills in ways that challenge their parents. Your preschooler is developing a sense of identity and personal agency and wants some control over things. But it is still important for parents to set limits on what they are allowed to do and where and when they can do it. They need their parents to help them learn how to get along with others, keep them safe, and let them know what is expected of them in different situations. They also need their parents to begin allowing them to have some autonomy and choices in their daily lives. These choices don't have to be complicated and can be kept simple, such as choosing to wear a dinosaur or Superman shirt or whether to have apple or orange juice. Choices help children understand that they are valued and important and that their ideas matter.

The practice of the bonus book came about because Amanda wanted to reward good behavior rather than always punishing her children for misbehavior. Because she knew that reading every day is important for kids and she also enjoyed this nightly routine, she didn't want to take away Mollie's bedtime book as a consequence of misbehavior. Instead, she created the bonus book, which gave Mollie an incentive to be good, listen, and follow simple household rules. Because she got the bonus book almost every night, it became part of their routine. This story illustrates something important to understand about preschoolers—that part of their development involves thinking and figuring out how to control their own lives. Mollie got to choose the books to read from a small shelf in her room and loved this special one-on-one time each night. Preschoolers are clever, and they understand, even at this age, quite a bit about how the world works. They can do simple math, even fractions, if using concrete examples—two halves of a sandwich (or a book) make a whole. They can communicate their feelings and desires. They understand others' feelings (though often need to be reminded), and they can play simple games with friends.

MILE MARKERS

As in the last chapter, we present developmental milestones, or mile markers, that can help you know what to expect at each age range in Table 4.1 (Berk, 2015). The preschool years can be some of the most rewarding times as a parent. Children start to make friends, enjoy playing with others, can have amazing conversations with adults, ask a lot of questions, and are constantly trying to figure out their world. Developmental researchers have called children in this period "little scientists" because children naturally want to discover why and how things work. When Caleb was 3, Amanda remembers him asking in the car one day, out of the blue, "How can God be in Heaven and in our heart?" Amanda was surprised by this complex philosophical question coming from her little boy, strapped into his car seat, but it was clear he had been pondering this for some time. She did her best to answer, realizing that giving a simple answer was all that was needed (God is everywhere at the same time) rather than getting into religious theology.

Three- and 4-Year-Olds

Children at this age are learning to think more logically and to make cause-and-effect connections. They see things as right and wrong, all

TABLE 4.1. Developmental Milestones in Early Childhood (Ages 3–5)

Age	Physical	Language	Thinking and learning	Social and emotional
3- and 4-year-olds	• Running, jumping, hopping, throwing, and catching become more coordinated • Can skip and gallop • Can draw simple pictures • Can use a fork and scissors • May not need a daytime nap	• Uses complex sentences and metaphors • Can adjust speech with different people (e.g., adults vs. younger siblings) • Can speak in multiple languages	• Understands cause and effect • Sorts objects into categories • Can count up to 10 • Is able to follow simple directions and rules • Can play simple games	• Labels and understands causes and consequences of emotions • Imitates adult behaviors, often in exaggerated ways (dress-up, shaving, cooking) • Can take the perspective of others • Has friends • Uses basic emotion regulation strategies
5-year-olds	• Can tie shoes • May start to lose baby teeth • Can use a knife to cut soft food • Can copy numbers and words • Uses adult pencil grip	• Knows the alphabet • Can read and spell simple words • Uses proper grammar most of the time • By age 6, has a vocabulary of about 10,000 words	• Writes their name • Memory improves • Can tell stories • Can count to 20 • Can reason about justice and fairness • Has an interest in how things work and basic science	• Likes to play with other children • Problem solving improves • Sense of right and wrong becomes more advanced • Ability to empathize increases • Moral development shifts from external rules to internal conscience

or nothing, and good and bad. Often at this age, children start to enjoy preschool, which can be a great way to learn how to interact with others. Three- and 4-year-olds love to play outdoors. They can run, jump, throw, and climb. They begin talking more like adults and can speak in complex sentences, even when learning multiple languages. Preschoolers are beginning to be able to take the perspective of others and label and understand emotions. They are also getting better at managing their emotions and can take a breath to calm down but still benefit from parents helping them understand their feelings and how to cope with them.

Five-Year-Olds

By age 5, most children start some type of formal schooling or organized learning program. Five-year-olds typically know the alphabet and can count to 10 or higher, and many can read and spell simple words. Their vocabulary ability to use language to express themselves continues to improve, and by age 6, they know about 10,000 words. They can use a pencil or crayon well and enjoy writing their name and short words. They are great storytellers but may stretch the truth a bit or get confused about what is real and what is imaginary. Children at this age start to have best friends and prefer certain playmates. Their ability to empathize improves, and they start to develop an internal sense of right and wrong.

BALANCING ACTS WITH PRESCHOOLERS

As we saw in Chapter 3, balanced parenting is a way of approaching parenthood that avoids extreme reactions to children's behavior and respects the needs of parents and other family members as well as the needs of the child. It is a mindset as well as a set of strategies that differ according to a child's age and developmental stage. For 3- to

5-year-olds, the world is opening up. Instead of playing mostly at home or in small group childcare settings, they may begin to attend preschool and kindergarten classes. They meet new children and adults, learning new skills and thinking new thoughts. Their curiosity matches their energy level. They begin to have strong preferences— expressing their likes and dislikes of certain foods, toys, games, activities, and people. These strong likes and dislikes can create conflicts between children and their parents, siblings, and playmates because they develop before the ability to cooperate, negotiate, or take other people's perspectives are fully developed (Mollie's skillful negotiations notwithstanding).

Parents have a great opportunity during these years to help children learn how to ask for what they want appropriately, share in their pleasure when they are able to obtain a desired result, and help them learn how to gain a measure of control over the emotions that sometime overwhelm them. Balanced parenting during the preschool years typically focuses on helping children have opportunities to make choices while maintaining enough parental control to keep them safe, healthy, and engaged in appropriate activities. For example, you don't want to let them choose whether to brush their teeth before bed, but you can give them a choice between using the bubblegum- or strawberry-flavored toothpaste. Our days are full of choices, and sharing the simple ones with children helps them feel like they have a bit of a say in what they do. They are less likely to make demands on the more complicated or consequential choices when they have opportunities to exert a little influence throughout their day. Another balancing act you may often encounter during the preschool years is learning how much monitoring or watchfulness is needed because children at this age are starting to play alone and with their siblings and friends.

Preschoolers can get completely engrossed in pretend play if they have a few basic props to fuel their imaginations. All is well until a parent suddenly realizes they are too quiet and checks in on the preschooler and their friend to discover that the pretend hairstylist is using real scissors to give her friend a not-so-pretend haircut. Jennifer's 4-year-old brother was once discovered shaving off his eyebrows when his mother had left her razor within reach. Childproofing is one way to allow children more autonomy without being overly watchful or intrusive. It is hard to overemphasize the importance of giving children opportunities to play on their own and with friends. Play is how young children learn about what they are able and not able to do physically.

Nearly 100 years ago, the famous Russian psychologist Lev Vygotsky studied children playing in preschools and concluded that "in play a child is always above his average age, above his daily behaviors; in play it is though he were a head taller than himself" (Vygotsky, 1978, p. 102). Why? Because when children are playing, they willingly control their actions, constraints that they might resist outside of play. And there is no pressure being put on them by adults. For example, when children pretend to have a tea party, they follow the social rules of taking turns, passing the pretend cookies, and making polite conversation with their stuffed animals. But there are no real cookie crumbs or actual "tea" or juice to spill, so they can focus on acting grown up and polite. When they play games, such as Simon Says, they are more likely to control their impulse to act until Simon says and can make themselves be still and quiet when playing hide and seek. Parents can be involved in playtime as long as they stay in their lane, letting children make the rules and follow their directions. And don't be surprised when the rules change mid-story!

Play is how children practice being sociable, too, beginning to understand the world around them and working through tough feelings. For example, one little 3-year-old we love knew that a future baby brother was growing in her mommy's tummy. In between using a pretend stethoscope to "hear" the baby's heartbeat in her mother's tummy and changing her baby doll's diapers, she pretended she had three babies in her own tummy, each with invented names and future personalities. Pretending to be a mom helped her welcome a new baby into her life. Balanced parenting allows children the freedom to play with only enough interference to ensure their safety. By controlling their own play, preschoolers learn to take the initiative to manage themselves and their environment rather than becoming overly dependent on others, fearful of acting on their own. This ability to initiate activities and interactions with others helps children develop a sense of purpose and character. It helps them develop the belief that "I am good" (see Table 4.2), and they begin to see that they are responsible for their actions and relationships.

Because preschoolers are beginning to understand how their thoughts, feelings, and actions affect others around them, this is an ideal time to start teaching them about being a person of character—acting and thinking in ways that will ultimately allow them to live a life of meaning and purpose. Parents can help their children develop character by recognizing, labeling, and making positive comments about their actions when they occur naturally in everyday life. In the activity at the end of Chapter 1, we presented a list of values and encouraged you to think about what you value in yourself, others, and your children.

When writing this book, we discovered a website and program that we like, The Virtues Project™ (de Moor, 2011). Psychologists

TABLE 4.2. Balanced Parenting During Early Childhood

Stage and age	Developmental challenges	Balanced parenting	Resilient child outcomes
Early childhood (3–5)	• Initiative versus fearfulness	• Exercising control versus giving choices	• Character (I am good)

in Canada began this global program, drawing on all the world's great wisdom traditions, to help parents and teachers raise children of compassion and integrity and promote personal healing in adults. It began with the idea that all children are born with the potential for these and other good qualities or "virtues," and when parents awaken these gifts of character, not only will the children and families be happier but the world will also become a more peaceful and joyful place. The programs they developed are being used by parents and teachers all over the world to help children learn how to express their feelings appropriately, act in harmony with others, and feel more confident. Research shows that too much vague praise—for example, saying "good job" or "way to go" all the time—actually lowers children's confidence (Brummelman et al., 2017). Nor is it effective to continually tell your child to "say you're sorry" or "use your words" multiple times a day. But teaching preschool children about specific virtues such as kindness, honesty, and helpfulness and how we use them in everyday life to get along helps them learn what behaviors we expect from them, how to express their feelings, and how to control their actions. It builds on their increasing understanding of how their behavior affects others, reduces conflict, and makes for happier homes and schools. Some specific strategies they have developed are described in Practical Tip 4.1: The Virtues Project™, and more information is included in the Resources section at the end of the chapter.

Practical Tip 4.1: The Virtues Project™

There are three ways to have a virtues conversation with your preschooler: (a) in the present, to acknowledge a virtue they are currently using; (b) about the future, to prepare them to use a virtue in an upcoming situation; and (c) about the past, to remind them when they forgot to use

(continues)

Practical Tip 4.1: The Virtues Project™ (*Continued*)

a virtue, how they could have done something differently, and how we talk about things that happened. When having a virtues conversation, there are three parts to include:

- use an opening phrase, drawing children's attention to what you're about to say;
- name the virtue, creating awareness of the many virtues they possess; and
- provide a few details about the situation, describing how the virtue was used or how it could be used.

Parents can keep a list of virtues on a poster on the wall or download cards online of virtues explained with pictures. Every day, parents can let the child pick a virtue so that parents can read what it says and think about a time that they used those virtues. For example, you might say, "Remember yesterday when we were eating ice cream? When you gave your little sister some of your ice cream after she dropped hers on the floor and was upset? You were being caring. Caring is looking for ways to be thoughtful and loving to others, just like you did." When parents see a virtue in action, they can say, "I appreciate your patience while we wait for your sister to be ready to go to the park." Parents can provide guidance for the future: "We will need to use friendliness today when we go to our friend's birthday party. There will be children you don't know, and it's good to play with new friends." Parents can also use a virtues conversation to correct or remind children when they forgot to practice a virtue and how they could have done something different: "I think you forgot to use courtesy today at Grandma's when you grabbed a cookie without asking. Next time remember to say please and thank you." Preschools and parents who have been using these strategies find that it only takes a bit of practice to stop for a second before responding to something their children have said or done, think about the virtue involved, and talk about it with their children. In fact, the preschools that have used it find that children use the virtues language and conversations with others when they are playing among themselves! (See Resources section for more information.)

A constant balancing act for parents at all ages is to meet children's needs while also taking care of themselves, but this can be especially tricky during the preschool years. Children's verbal skills are exploding, as is their need to understand and talk about the world. Preschoolers have often stopped napping, so a day with a preschooler is a day full of questions without time to rest or enjoy a quiet moment. Parents of preschoolers often protest that they would just like to be able to visit the bathroom alone without seeing little fingers waving under the door or hearing a little voice asking when they will come out. Preschoolers have more complex social and emotional needs than infants and toddlers, and parents sometimes need to recharge their own batteries after a day of helping their little ones manage their frustrations and worries. Between 3 and 5 years, children begin to ask questions about life and death, the differences they notice between boys and girls, and the reasons for all the "no's" or "not now" responses they hear daily. Questions such as "Why is the sky blue?" or "What happened to the dinosaurs?" can create opportunities for discoveries that are as fun for parents as for children.

It is tempting to let them sit with a screen or TV, but this should not be a habit. You may remember from Chapter 3 that the American Academy of Pediatrics recommends limiting children up to 5 years to 1 hour a day of screen time. They learn more by doing than by looking and will benefit more (and sleep better) if they've been involved in more active pastimes. Take advantage of playgrounds and museums, go for walks playing "I spy with my little eye," check out books from the library, and visit websites together that provide engaging answers to preschoolers' questions—activities that parents and children can enjoy together. As much fun as preschoolers can be, parents also need to make time to enjoy themselves away from their children, engaging in activities that help them be physically and mentally healthy and spending time with friends.

PARENTING WHEN YOU HAVE ACEs: MANAGING YOUR EMOTIONS

Parents of preschoolers may find themselves remembering things their parents said to them or did when they were this age that continue to cause them pain and difficulty. Preschoolers are full of energy, questions, likes and dislikes, and the desire to do things their way. When parents grew up in homes where their curiosity and preferences were ignored, ridiculed, or punished, it can be hard to react positively to their children when their children lose their temper because they can't have the Spiderman plate or refuse to stay in their bed because of monsters or ask "Why?" for the 20th time that afternoon. If the parent constantly heard an angry "Because I said so; now leave me alone" or were slapped for similar behaviors, these may be the reactions that most quickly come to mind.

Zooming In 4.1: Emotion Regulation

One of Amanda's areas of scientific expertise is the development of emotion regulation. In this box, she distills some of the most important things scientists have learned about emotion regulation. First, emotions are signals that tell us something in our environment may not be right or is not typical. Anger tells us that we may need to prepare for something not going our way, and sadness signals loss or disappointment. Instead of ignoring emotions, we need to recognize what they are telling us. There may be nothing wrong, no loss or real threat, but we need to process why we are feeling this way. If you are experiencing lots of negative feelings for no reason, it is a good time to seek professional counseling.

Second, we need to learn how to regulate both positive and negative emotions. Sometimes, when we are excited or happy about something, we may have to hold back our reactions so that we can keep on going with what needs to be done or not make others feel uncomfortable if they are not feeling as joyful. For example, you may be happy when your child wins

Zooming In 4.1: Emotion Regulation (*Continued*)

the spelling bee, but there are other children who were eliminated in the first round. Sometimes we need to watch our expressions of excitement in situations like this.

Third, emotion regulation is context- and culture dependent. What we mean by this is that regulating emotions depends on the situation. In some situations, it is okay to show anger, cry hysterically, or jump up and down. Part of growing up is realizing how to express and communicate emotions in specific situations. With close friends, we can be more open. At work, we often must manage our emotions and responses so we can get our jobs done and minimize conflict.

Fourth, there are some strategies for regulating emotions that are most effective. This includes more active strategies such as problem solving, reframing a situation so it is no longer negative (e.g., I am glad my daughter did not win the spelling bee because the next round is during our family vacation), or getting support from a friend or partner. When we can't change the situation that is making us feel bad, sometimes it is best to distract ourselves from the situation by doing something fun such as going to a movie with a friend or something healthy such as exercising at the gym. We want to avoid more negative strategies such as emotional eating, using drugs or alcohol to cope, ruminating about the situation, or lashing out at those around us. One of the best strategies for handling emotions is to take care of ourselves so that when we feel emotions, we are ready to handle them. Being overly tired or stressed makes it challenging for anyone to handle emotions and not overreact.

Finally, it's possible to manage a potentially emotional situation before it even happens. For example, you can avoid interacting with someone you know always upsets you or plan for how to manage a difficult situation. As we have said throughout this chapter, practice being calm to stay calm when things get stressful. Mindfulness is a great way to develop this skill.

In previous chapters, you learned that the first step in breaking the intergenerational cycle of adverse childhood experiences (ACEs) is to become aware of your childhood experiences—both positive and negative—and recognize the patterns in your family that continue to influence how you think, feel, and respond now that you are a parent. Awareness of these influences on us is a great start. The second step in breaking these cycles is to master the art of taking control of your emotions. Almost without exception, the most important thing that parents can do during the preschool ages is to learn how to control their emotional responses to their children's behavior. We have all heard the advice to stop and count to 10 or stop and take a deep, calming breath before reacting. It sounds easy, but when it's your 4-year-old having a meltdown at the grocery checkout counter because they're not getting candy, and everyone is looking at you as if you're the worst parent in town, it can be harder than you imagined. So how does one turn off the automatic angry, frustrated, and impatient responses that spring to mind instead of the calm and understanding responses that help children gain some control over their emotions?

The answer is by practicing being calm when there is no crisis, practice that actually creates new brain architecture—neural networks that link emotion centers with thinking and control centers in our brain, a practice that retrains our biological responses to stress. There are a number of ways to get this training. One of the most effective is through mindfulness-based programs. For example, the 8-week mindfulness-based stress reduction (MBSR) program developed by Dr. Jon Kabat-Zinn (2005) has trained tens of thousands of people to control their reactions to others—as well as their intrusive and destructive thoughts—by practicing simple breathing and movement techniques. Even a few months of MBSR and other mindfulness practices have been found to change the brain, creating new pathways in the brain that help you stay calm and focused when you might otherwise get upset (Davidson et al., 2003). Many mindfulness practices are available for free or at a nominal cost online (see Resources). Yoga is also a popular and widely available practice for changing one's response patterns and learning to master one's emotions.

There are many other ways that parents can learn how to gain control over their automatic responses to emotionally provoking situations. For example, in his book *The Body Keeps the Score,* psychiatrist Dr. Bessel van Der Kolk (2014) described how acting on stage, singing in a choir, and working with horses or other animals can provide opportunities for the body to recover from trauma. These activities help individuals who have experienced trauma gain control over their emotions by allowing the body to have "experiences that deeply and viscerally contradict the helplessness, rage, or collapse that result from trauma" (van Der Kolk, 2014, p. 3). When a parent can overcome their own emotional storm and find calm, they can provide the calm in which their preschooler can find shelter and learn how to manage their feelings.

Two additional strategies can help parents with preschoolers, especially parents with a history of ACEs. The first is to create rules, expectations, routines, and a childproofed physical environment. As we said in Chapter 3, creating safe places for your child to play prevents many opportunities for preschoolers to "get into trouble," situations where they could get hurt, break objects, or make undesirable messes. This allows children to take the initiative in their play and develop control over their actions without being overly watched or managed. For example, having a craft box with washable markers, colored paper, safety scissors, nontoxic glue, and other materials that they can use at the kitchen table allows them to play on their own while you are making dinner or feeding their little sibling.

The second strategy is a theme that will continue throughout the book: taking care of yourself. When her children were small, and she was working full time, Jennifer remembers a few times when she felt like someone who had donated so much blood that she had none left to circulate in her own body. Pay attention when you have that thought! It is a big, red, flashing warning light on your dashboard that will only cause more serious problems if ignored. When parents feel depleted, they can barely meet the normal, routine requirements of parenting, much less any emotional upsets of their preschoolers. It is a good time for early bedtimes for all, with some extra stories to get everyone settled. Or it is a good time to make an exception to screen time and have a favorite children's movie and pizza night with extra blankets on the couch. When even this is too much to manage, it is the time to call in reinforcements—asking your partner to cover for you while you head to a friend's house for a good pity party or asking the grandparents to take the little darlings for the night. And it is a great time to practice some yoga or mindfulness activities described earlier because they help our bodies, as well as our minds, recover (see Resources).

PARENTING STRATEGIES FOR BUILDING RESILIENCE

There are a number of strategies parents can use to encourage resilience during the preschool years. We encourage you to use strategies that work particularly well for children in this age range and will build skills that will last throughout development.

Being Part of the Family

One way to build character is for children to learn early on what it means to be part of a family, be responsible, and help around the house. Preschoolers can and should be expected to pick up their toys, make their beds, help to fold clothes, set the table, and do other simple chores around the house. Kids love using adult tools such as child-size brooms, dusters, and spray bottles. They like to do adult things, and this can be quite useful! One of the best ways to encourage helping behaviors is to set expectations through simple rules and routines (e.g., we put away toys after we play, we take our plates to the sink after we eat). Children love it when we praise them and acknowledge their help. When we praise children, it is important to be specific, and this encourages children to keep helping and feel good about what they are doing. For example, you might say, "I like how you clear your plate after dinner; it helps me to have all the dishes in the kitchen when I put them in the dishwasher."

Children this age love to sort and categorize things. Stacking dishes and sorting clothes can be fun activities for preschoolers. In a recent visit to her son's house, Jennifer was amazed to see that her son Zack had his preschoolers unloading the dishwasher. They sorted the silverware and utensils into the drawers like pros. They couldn't reach the upper cabinets, but they knew where the dishes went and stacked the clean dishes below the cabinets where they belonged, and mom or dad put them up later. Zack had created a routine that worked, and the children were proud they could help to do something that grown-ups usually do.

Part of getting ready for the day can be making the bed, brushing teeth, and getting dressed. Children this age can dress themselves, although they may need a little help. Preschool teachers know that cleaning up is much more fun with a silly song. Making things fun or like a game ("Let's see how fast we can put away all the blocks") increases participation and makes chores part of everyday routines that help the household run more smoothly.

Be an Emotion Coach

In the 1990s, Dr. John Gottman, who is well-known for his books and research on marriage, also studied how parents respond to children's emotions. He identified parents as emotion dismissing, emotion punishing, or emotion coaching (Gottman, 2011). Emotion-coaching parents, rather than emotion-dismissing or punishing parents, had children who were better at emotion regulation (managing their feelings) and coping with negative emotions such as anger and sadness (Snyder et al., 2013).

Children this age feel emotions strongly but do not yet have the skills to handle them alone. Parents and teachers can help when they act as emotion coaches, labeling the feeling, helping children to express feelings appropriately, figuring out what caused the feelings, and teaching them how to become calm after an emotional storm. Sometimes this can be as simple as saying, "It looks like you are angry. Yes? I know it is frustrating when your little sister knocks down your Lego towers." We want to encourage children to label and solve their problems with support. Asking questions such as "How did that make you feel?" and "What can you do differently?" encourages children to start handling emotions and problems on their own. Rather than punishing a child for feeling or expressing an emotion, we can explain that their reactions can either help solve a problem or make it worse—for example, "It is okay to be angry, but it is not okay to hit your sister. And besides, that doesn't seem to work! What else can you do? Maybe wait to build your towers while she is napping?"

Many children this age may be afraid of things such as monsters and the dark. Their developing imagination skills seem to go into overdrive while they are sleeping, and children are now able to remember those bad dreams or nightmares when they wake. It is important for parents to be reassuring and help children to work through their fears. Look under the bed and in the closet, and leave on a night-light if that helps. When children have nightmares, encourage them to tell you what happened and come up with a different, less scary ending to the dream. This might involve them getting away from something bad or being a hero and stopping the bad guy (Davis, 2008). Don't dismiss their feelings or overreact to them. Your child might be deathly afraid of spiders simply because someone else overreacted once to spiders. When they tell you they're afraid and think there are spiders in their bed, acknowledge their fear, check the covers, and assure them there are no spiders. Be firm but kind and calm. This is sometimes easier said than done but will make it more likely that your child will conquer those fears more quickly than if you dismiss or ignore them. Check out Zooming In 4.2: The Disappointing Prize.

Zooming In 4.2: The Disappointing Prize

Amanda has done research that illustrates ways that parents can help pre-schoolers handle emotions such as anger, sadness, and disappointment using a clever laboratory paradigm called the "disappointing prize task." In this study, while parents were completing surveys, children were asked to rank 10 prizes, from the best (most favorite) to the worst (least favorite), and were told that they would receive the best prize at the end of the visit. There were a variety of prizes in the box, such as bubbles, a slinky, and a matchbox car. There were also less appealing prizes, such as baby socks, broken sunglasses, and a rattle. After the parent and child did some activities in a room together, the experimenter came in and gave the child their prize in a decorated brown paper bag. The experimenter left the room, and when the child opened the bag, they discovered it was the worst prize. After several minutes, the experimenter came back into the room, explaining that they had made a mistake and gave the child the best prize.

Amanda's lab examined the video-recorded responses of the parents and children to see what parenting behaviors worked best to calm children. When parents shifted the child's attention away from the prize ("Look at the decorated bag!"), children tended to calm down quickly. Problem solving and thinking of ways to make the prize better ("Let's give the car to your baby brother," "We can put the baby socks on the cat!") also worked well, as long as the child bought into the suggestion and agreed it was a good idea. Physical and verbal comfort (e.g., patting the child's arm, saying it's okay) was helpful for most children, too. This study illustrates the importance of parents working with children to help them learn how to handle their feelings. Most important, parents who did not try to help their child manage their feelings had children with more emotional problems in school, such as aggression with peers currently and several years later.

Have Fun

This is one of the most fun times to be a parent! Children this age love to play, make messes, and be around other children. It is a great time to make blanket forts, camp in the backyard, and make messes in the kitchen when baking cookies or making play dough. Parenting in the moment, or mindful parenting (see Practical Tip 4.2: Mindful Parenting) is a great way to be fully present and play with your children during this stage. As mentioned previously, children learn through play. So having simple toys such as blocks, crayons, colored paper, dolls, and action figures allows children to be creative and have fun on their own or with others. Children also are energetic at this age. You may need to plan for an outside activity every day for active preschoolers. If they do not burn off energy, the rest of the day will be difficult for all.

This is a great time to enjoy parks; have playthings in your backyard, such as a swing or sandbox; and go to the library. Another fun activity for children this age is birthday parties. They are a great way for parents to meet other parents, and children love seeing other kids

---

Practical Tip 4.2: Mindful Parenting

Researchers at the University of Wisconsin and Pennsylvania State University developed a model of mindful parenting that is useful for parenting across all age groups but may be particularly useful with preschoolers (Duncan et al., 2009). Mindful parents are "in the moment" and focused on the parent–child relationship. They are not thinking about work, how their child got in trouble at school, or how their child's behavior will affect who they become as adults. They are fully present and accepting of what is happening in the moment. There are several strategies you can use to help become a more mindful parent:

- Listen with full attention to your child. This may involve getting down to the level of the child and sitting on the floor to look directly at your child's face.

Practical Tip 4.2: Mindful Parenting (*Continued*)

- Be accepting. Rather than judging the child or judging yourself for a behavior, simply notice what is happening in the situation and accept it for what it is.
- Be aware of your emotions and the child's. Label how you and the child are feeling and acknowledge any differences. But stay calm. It is difficult, but remembering you are the parent can sometimes help.
- Show compassion for you and your child. Parenting is a tough job! And it is hard to be a kid, too! It is okay if you make a mistake and raise your voice in anger. This happens to all of us. Simply acknowledge your anger and apologize for yelling.

Remember that no parent is always mindful and focused on their child, nor should they be. We have relationships with others to manage ("What did my boss mean when he said that today?"), bills to pay, and a thousand other worries that sometimes keep us awake at night. But try to find at least 10 to 15 minutes a day to spend with your child, temporarily blocking out these other thoughts, and give them your attention. Research has shown it's worth the effort.

outside of regular activities such as school. The parties do not have to be elaborate for the children to have fun. All kids love cake and ice cream and playing games such as hide and seek and freeze tag in the backyard.

Discipline Versus Punishment

In the Active Parenting program, a widely used parent education program created by Dr. Michael Popkin, parent educators talk about the difference between discipline and punishment (Popkin et al., 2017). Discipline comes from the word *disciple*, which means "student" or "to learn." Punishment, however, refers to pain or loss, retribution for misbehavior. Taking a more teaching approach to discipline is much more effective than simply punishment, especially in the long run. Parents want children to do the right thing because it is the right thing, not because they fear punishment from a parent. After all, parents will not always be there when children are making choices about right and wrong. This ties into character development, which is our resilient outcome during this stage. Preschoolers are primed for understanding why behaviors are helpful or hurtful, right or wrong because they are learning about how social interactions and relationships work at this age and how to treat others.

There are times when a toy needs to be taken away or a parent needs to speak in a stern voice to get a point across, especially when

---

Practical Tip 4.3: Disciplining Preschoolers

- **Set up a child-friendly environment where children know what is expected.** Children misbehave for many reasons, often to get attention or because they are bored. Try spending just 10 minutes of quality time playing with each child in the family every day. Have toys and activities available that children can play with on their own (e.g., blocks, art supplies).
- **Punishment should never be done in anger or desperation.** Have a discipline plan and stick to it. Try using reasoning and logical consequences whenever possible. If a child needs time to calm down, have a quiet place for the child to sit and take some calming breaths or look at a book. Rather than making this a time-out, make it a time-in, where the child is removed from a situation but has a space to regulate their behaviors and feelings. This may be alone time in a designated space, such as a child's room, and the parent may be present or not, depending on what works best for the child.
- **Positive discipline does not equal lax parenting.** When parents avoid yelling, spanking, and harsh punishment, it does not mean children are spoiled. When parents don't respond at all and let children run the show, that is lax parenting. When parents give children everything they want, that is spoiling a child. When parents teach their child right from wrong, that is positive discipline.

---

a child's safety is at risk ("Don't touch the stove; it will burn you"), but teaching children why a behavior is problematic and allowing for natural or logical consequences is the discipline approach most experts agree works best. For example, if a child won't share a toy with a friend, a parent can take it away for a while. That is a *logical consequence*. If a child leaves a toy outside in the rain, and it gets ruined, that is a *natural consequence*. When such things happen, it is important for parents to explain why it happened and talk about how to avoid such outcomes in the future. For example, a parent might say, "Oh no, you left your truck outside instead of putting it away inside. Now the wheels are rusted. Maybe we can fix it. But next time, remember to put toys back inside when you are finished playing with them unless they are outside toys." When parents respond like this, they are focusing on the behavior, not the child. If instead, parents say something such as, "That was a stupid thing to do. You should have known to put your toys away in case it rained," children feel bad about themselves rather than bad about a behavior that they can change in the future.

Another crucial part of being an effective parent is that parents should always avoid using harsh punishment—yelling, hitting, and spanking. Hundreds of studies have found that a more positive approach to discipline is best, leading to a better parent–child relationship and more positive outcomes such as moral reasoning, empathy, and helping behavior. In contrast, studies on spanking and harsh parenting have consistently found that these behaviors lead to more child aggression. Although not all children who are spanked will become aggressive, research has indicated that most of the effects of spanking on children are negative. After doing a thorough review of all the research on corporal punishment, Dr. Elizabeth Gershoff and her colleagues at the University of Texas concluded that:

> The strength and consistency of the links between physical punishment and detrimental child outcomes lead the authors

to recommend that parents should avoid physical punishment, psychologists should advise and advocate against it, and policymakers should develop means of educating the public about the harms of and alternatives to physical punishment. (Gershoff et al., 2018, p. 626)

This may be difficult for some parents, especially if they were raised in a home where parents spanked their children. Both Amanda and Jennifer were spanked as children because that was the primary disciplinary strategy most parents in Texas knew to use when they were children. But because Amanda and Jennifer learned about more effective ways to help children learn how to control their behavior (partly through studying child development!), they chose not to spank their own children. There is now more evidence for why parents should avoid spanking. We realize other discipline strategies may take some effort to learn and use, but we think they are worth it in the long run. If this is challenging for you or you want more information on positive discipline, find a parenting program in your community or see the Resources section at the end of this chapter.

PARENTING CHILDREN WHO HAVE A HISTORY OF ACEs

As we saw in Chapter 3, the same parenting strategies that work well for children without ACEs are good parenting practices for children with a history of ACEs. But children who have experienced trauma may behave in ways that require us to develop more patience and practice remaining calm. Children with a history of adversity may have more difficulties managing their emotions than other children. Their ability to control their impulses may be slower to develop. Our friends and colleagues in the Department of Pediatrics at the University of Oklahoma studied the effects of both adverse and protective childhood experiences on the social and emotional development of preschoolers across the United States (Yamaoka & Bard, 2019). They discovered that six simple daily activities protected children from the negative effects of ACEs. These six positive parenting practices were:

- having family meals together;
- going on outings to places such as parks, museums, zoos, or family gatherings;
- telling stories or singing songs;
- reading;
- playing with peers; and
- limiting screen and television time.

Children with ACEs who did not have these activities had delayed social and emotional development. But we think it even more important that they found that the absence of these positive parenting practices was as harmful to children's development as having four or more ACEs. This is a remarkable finding, given the powerful negative effects of ACEs, and it highlights the equally powerful effects of good parenting practices.

In addition to engaging in positive activities with children, parents also need to have rules and limits. You may notice that when your children come back from a weekend at the grandparents' house, they have to relearn the rules. At Grandma's, children often get to eat lots of sugary food that they may not get at home, watch movies, stay up late, and do fun activities. When they come home, you may have to go into what we call "boot camp" mode. You have to be extra firm and consistent with bedtime and snacks for a few days before the kids get back into their routines and remember the rules of their home. But kids benefit from having strong relationships with other family members (having other adults to count on is a protective and compensatory experience [PACE]!), and parents often need a break from meeting the continuous needs of small children. If you think the differences in rules and routines are more than your child can handle, talk with the grandparents or other family members your child visits to find ways to be more consistent. The balance of allowing children freedom and limiting behavior naturally ebbs and flows. Sometimes things at home will get too lax, and children will start running the show, especially when parents are tired or stressed. It is important for parents to get back on track and enforce limits and expectations with logical and natural consequences during these times. It may take a few days, but talk with your children about what to expect and why things are changing, and be consistent once you commit to a new routine.

Another important parenting strategy for children with a history of ACEs is to make sure that their basic daily needs are met. Remember our discussion in Chapter 2 about the importance of protective and compensatory experiences (PACEs) for helping both children and parents recover from ACEs? Are they getting enough physical activity? Are they getting enough sleep? Are they eating healthy foods and not too much sugar? Children in this age range need lots of activity and lots of sleep. It is recommended that children aged 3 to 5 get 3 hours of activity a day, and 1 hour should be very active, including running, jumping, or playing sports. In terms of sleep, 3- to 5-year-olds need 10 to 13 hours of sleep each night. Having a bedtime routine and getting children to bed at 7:00 or 8:00 gives children the sleep they need and gives parents time for themselves. This is a great goal for families to work toward if children are not already used to early bedtimes.

You might want to make a note for a few days about other PACEs. Do they get opportunities to play alone and with others? Do they have opportunities to draw or paint, sing and dance, and learn about the world? Do they know they are loved, even when they misbehave or disappoint others? While all children (and parents) benefit from having PACEs in their lives, the PACEs that are particularly helpful to preschoolers are those that help them learn about the world; how to play, share, and care about others; and how to express and manage their feelings. For example, the PACEs related to friendship are important, both in one-on-one play and also in small groups. Because they need to be active, PACEs related to movement, such as gymnastics, dance, and beginner sports activities, are good for children. Going to preschool and prekindergarten classes helps them prepare for school and also satisfies their curiosity and interest in the world. It also opens up opportunities to meet new friends and new adults and gain new skills.

As we mentioned in Chapter 3, it is always advisable for parents to ask for help when they need it. Look around for resources in your community, or talk with your pediatrician or nurse, staff at the childcare center your child attends, or friends and family members. When children this age have already experienced abuse or neglect, they often have difficulty forming attachments and trusting others. It takes time and patience from caregivers to build back trust. They may also be overly friendly with strangers or not come to a parent when they need help or comfort. Consistently being there for the child, being responsive to their needs, and helping them feel safe builds trust over time.

All parents should have conversations with their children about safety at this age. Specifically tell children they can talk with you about anything that makes them feel worried, unsafe, or scared. Let them know that they should tell you if someone makes them feel uncomfortable. You may find it helpful to talk with your children about "good and bad touch." What is important is that children understand no one should ever touch their genitals or "private parts" and that if a strange adult ever approaches them, they should get help from an adult that they know and never get in a car or go anywhere with a stranger.

KEY TAKEAWAYS

The following are some of the main themes from this chapter to remember as you continue on your parenting journey:

- Become a master at recognizing and managing your emotions. Take a moment to become calm before responding to nonemergency situations. Practice being calm in the face of emotions using mindfulness, yoga, or other techniques (see Resources).
- Create a safe place for your preschooler to play, with simple hands-on toys such as plastic or wooden blocks, art supplies, board books, and pretend toys (e.g., child-sized kitchen utensils and pretend food, dolls, action figures). Make this a place where children can access toys on their own, and you can check in regularly but do not have to supervise every minute. This encourages children to choose activities.
- Kids this age love to play with other children, and you will benefit from adult time, too! Enroll your child in a quality preschool program and get to know other parents, or join a playgroup in your neighborhood. Going to the park, the library, and birthday parties can be fun for parents as well as their kids.
- Involve your preschooler in simple household chores, such as folding laundry, putting away the silverware from the dishwasher, or clearing the dishes after dinner. This can be the start of good household habits, and children this age love to do adult-like things.

- Have routines. This is important at all ages but especially during early childhood. Continue to read to your child at bedtime, letting your child choose the book(s). Having a routine with time for physical activity and plenty of sleep is helpful for everyone in the family, too.
- Use positive discipline strategies and be an emotion coach. Preschoolers struggle with managing their emotions, and it helps parents support them and talk through feelings and how to handle them. Instead of yelling or spanking your child, use logical and natural consequences and agree on simple rules your preschooler can remember and understand.

ACTIVITY: YOU ARE HERE

On your parenting journey, you have set some goals and have a destination in mind: a calm, loving home that helps children become good people when they are grown. Now, take a minute to think about where you are now.

- What am I doing well as a parent? What do I like most about my preschooler? What do I enjoy most about parenting at this age?
- Can I stop for a moment and think about how to respond when my child misbehaves? Am I labeling their feelings and actions? Have I tried using the language of virtues to help them understand their feelings and behaviors?
- Do I provide opportunities for them to make choices or play on their own, just monitoring occasionally?
- Where are you in terms of taking care of yourself? Do you make time for some routines that replenish your reserves of energy and patience? Do you do things just for fun? Do you have support from others and accept help when it's offered?

- Where are you in terms of balancing choice and control? Have you created a safe play environment for your preschooler? Do you create opportunities for your preschooler to make simple choices? Take a few minutes to write down your ideas on where you are with this balancing act and some things you might do differently.
- What PACEs does your child already have? What PACEs would you like to add next? What PACEs do you have for yourself to keep your energy and mood stable during the preschool years? What PACEs would you like to have? Now take a few minutes to write on a calendar or a piece of paper the PACEs for yourself and your child that you will add in the coming weeks and how you will go about it.

ACTIVITY: MINDFUL MEDITATIONS

One of the most important ways to be a parent who raises strong, happy, and resilient children is to take control of our emotional responses. When parents make mistakes, it is often because strong emotions negatively influenced their thoughts or actions. Fear and anger are two emotions that often get in the way of seeing situations clearly, causing reactions that are later regretted. Research has shown that the way to gain control over our emotions whenever they occur is to practice staying physically and emotionally calm using mindful meditations. There are many resources to help you begin a mindfulness practice, but the key word is *practice*. Mindfulness—the ability to stay calm and nonjudgmental and control one's reactions—is not learned from a book. It is learned by spending a little time every day or two practicing. One meditation we think is especially helpful for busy parents of preschoolers is the following loving-kindness meditation. Find a quiet time when you will not be interrupted for a few minutes, and try it. We recommend listening to the audio of this guided meditation at either of the following links:

https://ggia.berkeley.edu/practice/loving_kindness_meditation
https://mindworks.org/blog/lovingkindness-meditation-a-daily-script/

Other mindfulness meditations from Dr. Jon Kabat-Zinn include

https://www.youtube.com/watch?v=15q-N-_kkrU
https://www.youtube.com/watch?v=1H2Cgc60UlU

RESOURCES

Toilet Training

Gomi, T. (2020). *Everyone poops*. Chronicle Books.

Practical tips for parents: https://kidshealth.org/en/parents/toilet-teaching.html

Virtues

Popov, L. K. (1997). *The family virtues guide*. Plume.
The Virtues Project: https://www.virtuesproject.com
Parenting and family articles: https://www.greatergood.berkeley.edu

Mindfulness and Mindful Parenting Books

Clarke-Fields, H. (2019). *Raising good humans: A mindful guide to breaking the cycle of reactive parenting and raising kind, confident kids*. New Harbinger.
Kabat-Zinn, J. (2016). *Mindfulness for beginners: Reclaiming the present moment—and your life*. Sounds True.
Williams, M., & Shiels, K. (2017). *101 mindfulness games for happy minds: For children aged 3–7*. Early Impact Training.

Disciplining Without Hitting or Spanking

Faber, J., & King, J. (2017). *How to talk so little kids will listen: A survival guide to life with children ages 2–7.* Scribner.

Popkin, M., Morris, A. S., Slocum, R., & Hubbs-Tait, L. (2017). *Active parenting: First five years parent's guide.* Active Parenting.

Siegel, D. J., & Hartzell, M. (2013). *Parenting from the inside out: How a deeper self-understanding can help you raise children who thrive* (10th ed.). Penguin.

Parenting to Promote Positive Development

Dweck, C. (2007). *Mindset: The new psychology of success.* Ballantine Books.

Galinsky, E. (2010). *Mind in the making: The seven essential life skills every child needs.* Harper Collins.

Gottman, J., & DeClaire, J. (2011). *Raising an emotionally intelligent child.* Simon & Schuster.

Shulman, M., & Mekler, E. (1994). *Bringing up a moral child: A new approach for teaching your child to be kind, just, and responsible.* Doubleday.

Shure, M., & DiGeronimo, T. F. (1996). *Raising a thinking child: Help your young child to resolve everyday conflicts and get along with others.* Gallery Books.

CHAPTER 5

MIDDLE CHILDHOOD: BALANCING LIMITS AND INDEPENDENCE

When Jennifer was in the first grade, the philharmonic orchestra in the West Texas town of Abilene put on an afternoon concert just for elementary school children. This concert is one of Jennifer's favorite childhood memories. The whole experience felt magical. She and her classmates got on the bus—she normally walked to school, so the bus was an adventure alone—and filed into the auditorium. They sat down in plush red seats, the lights dimmed, and the soaring opening notes of George Gershwin's Rhapsody in Blue *filled the space. When Jennifer heard the piano solo, she was hooked. It was a life-changing moment. Jennifer went home and begged her parents for piano lessons.*

Only when she was an adult did she realize the sacrifices her parents made to fulfill this request. They found a piano teacher two blocks away so she could walk to her weekly lessons. They rented a piano for several months to see if this was the passing fancy of a 7-year-old or a real commitment. When they realized that she was serious about it, they bought a beautiful Kimball studio piano "in installments" during the age before credit cards. The piano was placed in the small living room that no one used except when guests came, where she could practice without distractions. When she learned a three-note song at her first lesson, her father proudly called the neighbors in to hear her play it. Her mother regularly told her that she would rather listen to her play the piano than have her help with the dishes, making practicing seem less like a chore. Every year there was an evening recital. And every year, on the afternoon of the recital, there was a corsage with a note from her father waiting for Jennifer in the refrigerator when she came home from school. One of her happiest memories is finally playing the piano solo from Rhapsody in Blue *at one of the recitals, with her parents beaming in the audience.*

MILE MARKERS

Middle childhood is an important time for children's physical, social, and cognitive development. By the end of the first grade, children should be able to read short sentences and spell simple words. By the second grade, most children will be reading simple books on their own, and the transition from "learning to read to reading to learn" is taking place. By third grade, it is essential that children can read; otherwise, they will continue to face academic challenges throughout schooling and possibly later in life. Consider finding a program or a retired teacher who tutors children in the evenings or on weekends if your child is still struggling to read after the second grade. You may find traditional strategies of going over sight words and math facts on flash cards helpful during this stage. Experts agree that combining hands-on learning with more conventional strategies of learning phonics and memorizing math facts works well. It is important to enrich the more traditional methods with experiences that bring math and reading concepts to life.

Parents should make sure their children are making adequate progress in school and be their advocates when they need additional support or assistance. If your child is having difficulties in school, this is a good time to check whether their struggles are due to attention-deficit/hyperactivity disorder (ADHD) or other learning disabilities such as dyslexia, dysgraphia, or auditory processing disorders. These and other learning problems can be addressed once they are diagnosed and incorporated into children's educational plans. It is also important to note that children who are experiencing or have experienced trauma are sometimes misdiagnosed with ADHD or other learning disabilities because of the effects of stress on the brain. It is critical to diagnose and treat underlying causes as well as symptoms to ensure children's long-term success and well-being.

Physical changes are taking place, too! It is in kindergarten or first grade when children lose their first tooth. This can be an exciting time, and many first-grade classrooms have tooth charts where they graph the number of teeth collectively lost by the class. The tooth fairy can be fun during this time because children still enjoy make-believe and fantasy play. As children get older, parents will have to decide what to tell children about make-believe characters such as Santa Claus, the tooth fairy, and the Easter Bunny. There is no one right way to do this, but as children age, it is important to answer their questions honestly.

As discussed later in this chapter, many children, especially girls, start puberty during middle childhood. The average age for *menarche*, the age of the first menstrual period, has been steadily declining for decades. In the United States, it is around age 12, with about 10% around age 10 (Eckert-Lind et al., 2020). The early signs of puberty appear for most girls between 9 and 11 with breast buds. For boys, puberty typically starts around 11, with the testicles growing and the start of pubic hair. Being an early developer may be difficult for children because it puts them out of step with their peers. For example, if your daughter enters puberty around 10, she will need your support in learning to handle the practical complications of menstrual bleeding and cramps long before her friends and peers start talking about it or are similarly concerned. She may also be faced with unwanted attention from older boys because her physical development will make her appear older than she is. Make sure you talk with your children before you think it's time, so they are prepared whenever they enter puberty and can be considerate if and when their friends do. (See Table 5.1 for the developmental milestones of middle childhood; Berk, 2015.)

Children are also developing more complex images of themselves, or self-concepts, and enjoy trying a variety of activities at this age. Parents should encourage children to join a variety of different clubs and organizations and talk about what happens at school and during activities. It is important for parents to acknowledge successes and be encouraging when children experience challenges or failures. Ask children what they are looking forward to each week. Friendships are becoming more influential, and children care about being accepted by their peers. Having "playdates" and getting to know other families can be helpful for parents and enjoyable for all.

Children this age love rules, but they begin seeing the world as more complex than they did as preschoolers. They understand that people do not always show their true feelings, that having information and experiences can affect the decisions people make, and that not everyone has the same information or life experiences. Their sense of fairness and justice is starting to develop, and moral reasoning becomes more advanced (more on this in Chapter 6). This is a great time to start having conversations about what is fair, what is going on in the world and their communities, and why different people are treated differently. More information on helping children deal with racism and discrimination is presented later in this chapter; it is a struggle for many kids this age (see the Resources section at the end of the chapter).

BALANCING ACTS IN MIDDLE CHILDHOOD

Balanced parenting during middle childhood involves maintaining a healthy balance between setting reasonable limits and allowing children more independence, being overly involved versus not involved

TABLE 5.1. Developmental Milestones in Middle Childhood (Ages 6–11)

Age	Physical	Language	Thinking and learning	Social and emotional
6 to 8-year-olds	• Permanent teeth gradually replace baby teeth • Writing is easier to read • Drawings are more detailed • Can play sports and games with rules	• Learns about 20 words a day • Conversations become more sophisticated	• Transitions from "learning to read to reading to learn" • Can use memory strategies such as repetition and rehearsal • Can do addition and subtraction up to 20 • Can count to 100 by ones, twos, fives, and 10s • Can write and recognize numbers up to 100 • Knows the values of coins	• Understands that others have different perspectives due to different information • Knows that people can experience multiple emotions at once • Understands that people can hide their true feelings • Can understand intentions • Wants to be liked and accepted by their friends

(continues)

TABLE 5.1. Developmental Milestones in Middle Childhood (Ages 6–11) (Continued)

9 to 11-year-olds	• Girls start growth spurt (2 years before boys) • Reaction time improves and affects performance in sports • Females have breast buds and pubic hair • Around 11 in males, testicles become bigger and pubic hair grows at the base of the penis	• Uses words more precisely • Understands double meaning of words, metaphors, humor • Stories become more detailed and involved	• Understands money and change • Can read a map • Can do multiplication and division, eventually long division and three-digit multiplication • Understands fractions • Can estimate and round numbers	• Friends become more important • Is more aware of their body • Can regulate and cope with emotions on their own, using different strategies • Understands personal choice and basic rights • Is more selective about friends • Is more aware of gender stereotypes

enough, and, as always, being focused on their own versus their children's well-being. Middle childhood gives parents a change of pace from the more intensely emotional and often demanding needs of 3- to 5-year-olds. Children between the ages of 6 and 11 still have much to learn, but they are better at managing their feelings and can channel their energy into their developing interests. As we saw in the Mile Markers section, they are getting a handle on the rules in their world—in games, at home, and at school. At school, they are starting to acquire more knowledge, gain new skills, and compare themselves with others. One of the goals for parents during these middle childhood years is to help their children develop a sense of competence—a belief that with persistence and practice, they can do the things they need to do (Harter, 2015).

Zooming In 5.1: Self-Concept and Self-Esteem

Psychologist Susan Harter (2015) was one of the first to show that children begin to develop their sense of self and self-esteem—how they think and feel about themselves—during elementary school. Children begin to ask themselves questions such as "Who am I?" "How do I fit in?" and "What am I good at?" During the early grades, they tend to exaggerate their abilities because they don't know yet what they can do, and they haven't had much experience seeing how their abilities compare with other children their age. But by the end of elementary school, children have a more accurate and relatively stable sense of self-worth. Dr. Harter found that children's overall self-esteem is based on how well they judge themselves relative to their peers in five areas: (a) social, (b) academic, (c) behavioral, (d) athletic, and (e) physical appearance.

Using Diana Baumrind's (1971) definition of parenting, which includes being nurturing and communicative, with age-appropriate expectations and consequences, Dr. Harter found that authoritative parents have children

(continues)

Zooming In 5.1: Self-Concept and Self-Esteem (*Continued*)

with higher overall self-esteem. Parents can also help children develop a positive self-concept by encouraging and supporting them in the areas where they have interests and talents and attaching less importance to areas where their abilities are more limited. Self-worth often decreases for girls when they enter puberty and adolescence, especially if their overall self-esteem is heavily based on their perceived physical appearance. Culture and peers begin to have a greater influence on children's self-worth, and parents can help by drawing attention to the unhelpful or damaging messages that children are exposed to through the media, other kids, or other adults. Parents can help them base their self-esteem on their developing skills and areas of competence rather than focusing on their physical appearance, material possessions, or other superficial qualities prevalent on social media and in popular culture. Parents are better able than their children to help them base their self-worth on their strengths, highlighting the areas that reflect their values and goals.

Children develop a sense of competence by discovering activities they enjoy so much that they are motivated to put in the time and energy that will allow them to do well. Feeling competent is the inner reward children experience when they have stuck with a new task, working through their frustration at not being able to do it perfectly at first. When children try out a new sport or hobby but lack the interest, support, or perseverance to gain the requisite skills to enjoy it, there are several possible outcomes. The first outcome is when they decide that a particular interest was just not for them after all. No worries—they go on to try another one. This is fine when it happens occasionally. But when children give up too frequently or easily, a second outcome is that they doubt themselves, question whether they can do anything well, and are reluctant to try new things in the future. The third outcome is to problem solve—figure out whether there was something they could have done differently.

Parents can influence which outcome occurs. First, they can provide support by helping children have time to practice and the resources needed to learn. Jennifer's parents provided a great example of this when they supported her interest in learning to play the piano. Second, they can help children decide whether they are really interested in something or whether a different sport, interest, or activity would be a better fit for them. In helping children discover their interests and goals, using a balanced parenting approach helps you avoid putting too much pressure on children to persist at one extreme or being too uninvolved or unsupportive at the other extreme. (Table 5.2 summarizes balanced parenting in middle childhood.)

Balanced parenting also helps parents set the limits for their 6- to 11-year-old children, allowing them the independence to develop their unique interests. We saw in Chapter 2 that children of all ages (and adults) benefit from physical activity and hobbies. During middle childhood, many of these interests emerge. As children become aware of the variety of pursuits and activities available, their interests become more distinct. Sometimes these interests are almost irrepressible, and children will pursue them independently of their

TABLE 5.2. Balanced Parenting in Middle Childhood (Ages 6–11)

Stage and age	Developmental challenges	Balanced parenting	Resilient child outcomes
Middle childhood (6–11)	• Perseverance versus self-doubt	• Establishing limits versus encouraging independence	• Competence (I can do things)

parents, seeking out resources through their school, the library, or other community sources. However, most of the time, parents need to provide their children with opportunities to help them find ways to learn about different potential activities. This may include signing them up for after-school classes at school, the YMCA, or other community organizations that provide after-school programs.

The challenge for parents is to decide how much independence they are comfortable allowing their children to have and where to place limits. For a small fee, Jennifer's children attended after-school programs at their public elementary school and could choose the programs they wanted, learning sign language, baking cookies from scratch, and doing art projects. Scouting is another way children can learn and practice new skills in a safe environment. They can be independent within the limits of the program. Parents who want to be more involved can volunteer as scoutmasters or help coach their children's sports teams.

Volunteering and being involved with children's groups help parents feel more comfortable about their children having activities away from home. It also helps them get to know their children's friends and their friends' parents. Getting to know the parents of your children's friends and schoolmates is a good way to be informed about who your children are spending time with when they are with their friends. This is the age when best friends form, when children play at their friends' houses and go to sleepovers. When you know their friends' parents, it is much easier to have conversations about the limits on their behavior. For example, at their house, are your two first-graders allowed to play outdoors in the front yard or only in the backyard? Can they walk to the corner store and back for an after-school snack? Can they walk home from the school bus stop together? These decisions will depend on parents' perceptions of their children's maturity and trustworthiness and the risks involved in any of the activities. And because these perceptions change as your children and their activities change, if you have good relationships with the parents of your children's friends, you will feel comfortable having those conversations. In fact, many parents find that these friendships with the parents of their children's friends are among the most enduring friendships they have.

Good parenting at every age requires finding the right balance between taking care of yourself and taking care of your child. Maintaining one's physical and mental health during middle childhood can be challenging—not because children are so demanding, but because family life often becomes more complicated as children get older. As children are involved in more activities, parents may spend more time in the car driving their kids to soccer practice and games, music lessons, dance classes, friends' houses, scouts—the list can go on and on. Parents and children can both become overwhelmed if they have too many outside activities. A rule of thumb many parents use is to allow only one physical activity and/or one hobby during the school year. This ensures that your 10-year-old has time at home to do homework, feed the dog, and spend time with the family while also playing on a soccer team and taking piano lessons. Carpooling with other families can be a help. You may find yourself spending several afternoons a week like an airport traffic controller, keeping track of where your child is and who they are with while juggling Zoom meetings at work.

Single parents need to take special care to create time for themselves. Sometimes this takes a little creativity as well as perseverance. Jennifer once knew a woman who was able to go back to college as a single parent with two school-age children while working on the assembly line of an auto plant because of an ingenious childcare solution she and her neighbors devised. The moms in this apartment complex got together and decided they could all go back to college or trade school and improve their economic futures if they helped each other with after-school and evening childcare. Each night during the school week, one of the four single moms took a turn watching the others' children. While the kids did their homework, had dinner, and played in one of the apartments, the other moms went to class and studied. By the time Jennifer met her, this woman had become a doctor, and her two children had graduated from college. What a testament to the power of friendship and cooperation!

PARENTING WHEN YOU HAVE ACEs: RECOGNIZE YOUR COPING HABITS FROM CHILDHOOD

As in other chapters, we provide tips and information on parenting with your history of adverse childhood experiences (ACEs). The most important thing parents can do to help their children be resilient is to build their own resilience, working through the enduring effects of their childhood trauma. When parents have a history of ACEs, random events in their children's lives can bring about unwanted thoughts and feelings that can negatively affect their parenting. These feelings may seem to come out of nowhere, especially if the trauma or abuse was pushed out of their conscious memory as a child and never dealt with. Trauma memories lose their power when they are brought to the surface and talked about with someone who is able to listen and be supportive—a trustworthy friend or professional counselor.

When we look at childhood trauma memories as adults, our goal is not to relive them, dwell on them, or make them a central part of our identity. Rather, we look back on them from the vantage point of being an adult now. As many children do, we may have blamed ourselves for being abused or neglected. But as adults, we can look back and realize that our childhood selves were not to blame. Adults can more easily recognize that their childhood selves were doing their best to survive difficult situations with the limited resources available to them. They can see themselves as survivors rather than victims. The first step, which we talked about in Chapters 2 and 3, is to take a courageous and compassionate look back at one's childhood and the family history of adversity and resilience and identify ghosts and angels in the nursery—past experiences from childhood. The second step, as discussed in Chapter 4, is to learn how to regulate your emotions to stay calm with your child and be a mindful parent. You're now ready for the next step.

Childhood Adaptations to ACEs (ChAACEs)

The third step of breaking the intergenerational cycle of ACEs is to recognize the adaptations, or survival strategies, that allowed your childhood self to cope with ACEs or other traumatic events. Researchers and psychologists who study the effects of childhood trauma or mistreatment have identified common coping strategies that children use to manage the challenges of living in situations where their physical and emotional needs are not being met (Osmanoglu, 2019). Some of these adaptations are positive ways to cope with stress and hardship. For example, being physically active, seeking help from other adults, focusing on schoolwork, or engaging in other positive activities have both short-term and long-term positive effects. Other responses have short-term benefits, given the specific situation at the time but are not good long-term strategies. For example, when children's parents are unable to take care of them because of alcohol or other substance abuse, they may learn ways to keep teachers or others from knowing what is going on to prevent them from feeling sorry for them or alerting the authorities. They become adept at maintaining a positive but false image, making excuses, and keeping others from knowing too much about them or their home life.

Children may even try to fill the role of the parent for themselves and their siblings. As adults, these children often find it difficult to stop portraying an image that everything is fine even when it's not, preventing them from genuinely connecting with others and accepting support when it is offered. Children of parents with mental illness often learn to ignore their own needs or negative feelings because their parents are frequently unable to attend to or react to them appropriately. As adults, they may have difficulties expressing feelings appropriately because they didn't learn how to while growing up. They learn not to trust others because their parents' promises were often forgotten. As effective as these childhood adaptations may have been at helping children cope at the time, they are usually not helpful when carried into adulthood or when they are used in place of more flexible and mature coping strategies.

The challenge for parents with ACEs who are now trying to raise healthy, resilient children is to recognize the coping strategies they used as children and decide which ones may still be beneficial and which ones are not. In the next chapter, we will talk about how to let go of past strategies that are no longer helpful and how to keep the ones that are working. The activity at the end of the chapter provides an opportunity to reflect on the survival skills you used as a child experiencing stress and adversity and start to think about whether they are still beneficial to you.

PARENTING STRATEGIES FOR BUILDING RESILIENCE

There are many strategies to help build resilience in school-age children. These reflect the balance between being involved and also letting children develop independence.

Support School Success

Parent involvement in children's schooling is one of the best predictors of success in school. Parents need to attend parent–teacher conferences and stay aware of how their children are doing in school. Online resources such as classroom grade books make this easier, but talking with a teacher about your child's strengths and struggles is invaluable. Having a dedicated time and space for children to do homework is helpful for kids, too. This can be at the kitchen table while making dinner or when children get home and have a snack. Schedules may vary because of other activities. If children are in an after-school program, that is often a good time to get schoolwork done. Children benefit from parents checking in and being available to support them by helping them practice for a spelling test or go through their math facts. Before bed is a good time for children to read to their parents. You may find that alternating between reading a chapter of a more advanced book to them and then listening to them read aloud one of their own books is a good practice. As their reading improves, you can take turns reading the pages of a book.

Many parents find it difficult to be involved in their children's schooling because of their own negative experiences with school. Often, parents do not even realize that their fears and anxieties from traumatic school experiences are limiting their ability and willing-ness to be involved in their children's schooling. It can be difficult to overcome this, but talking about it with a close friend or partner can help. Acknowledging the past makes it easier to move forward. Most teachers are eager to meet the parents of their students, and they are typically warm and inviting. Another strategy is to bring a friend to a teacher conference so you are not alone, and all primary caregivers should try to attend if possible.

Attending events such as field days, holiday parties, and occa-sional school lunches is a good way to be involved. When Jennifer's son Zack was in elementary school, he told her she should come to lunch on Fridays because they served gumbo, and it was delicious. With an invitation like that, how could she refuse? The noise was deafening, but Zack loved having her sit with him at lunch. She loved getting to know his friends and teacher better (and the gumbo was terrific). Most kids enjoy having parents or grandparents come to lunch at school.

Dropping off kids at school is often another way that parents can stay connected, especially when they are unable to get away from work during the day. Being seen by your children's teachers and peers can help reduce the chances that your child will be picked on or bullied by anyone and make it more likely that teachers or other school personnel will feel comfortable contacting you. Small problems are much easier to solve before they become big problems, and you want to encourage the school staff to let you know if your child hasn't turned in their homework for a few days or has started eating alone away from friends. Be sure to check with the school's front office to get instructions on how and when you and other caregivers can come to school and follow any of their protocols for visitors.

Practical Tip 5.1: Bullying

Unfortunately, many children experience bullying at school and may be especially vulnerable when they are not part of the majority culture. *Bullying* is typically defined as ongoing aggressive behavior that involves a power imbalance. This can involve physical or verbal aggression. Sometimes bullying can be relational (gossiping, excluding others from groups), particularly among girls. These days, a great deal of bullying occurs online. It is important for parents to talk about bullying, and be aware that it may be occurring at your child's school. Children can be involved as a victim of bullying, a bystander, or a bully. Sometimes, bullies are also victims. When having a conversation about bullying, talk about the importance of standing up for others.

Often, if bullies are not encouraged, the behavior will stop. Bystanders have an important role and can make a difference by supporting the victim and calling out the bullying as mean, not right, or hurtful. For the victims,

> **Practical Tip 5.1: Bullying (*Continued*)**
>
> role-playing works well. Have kids role-play what might happen and how they can respond (e.g., walk away, tell the bully to stop, get the teacher). Children typically do not want to "tattle" on others, but often teachers need to get involved. This is where an email, phone call, or text to the teacher from a parent can be helpful and make a big difference. If you think your child may be bullying others, talk with a school counselor. Figuring out why the bullying is occurring is important; address the problem directly by talking about it and checking in regularly.

Encourage a Variety of Activities

Middle childhood is a time when parents and children can enjoy many activities together. Parents may enjoy attending their children's softball games, school concerts, or end-of-year awards programs. What is fun but sometimes hard work is volunteering to help with your children's clubs and events. Helping to coach a soccer team, planning and going on scout camping trips, or assisting with school parties are great ways for parents to be involved and get to know their children's friends, teachers, and other parents. Children will have plenty of time to specialize in a sport or type of art at later ages. This is a time for exploration and fun!

In the 1980s, Dr. Howard Gardener developed the theory of multiple intelligences (Gardner, 2006). Much like Dr. Susan Harter, whose research we described in Zooming In 5.1: Self-Concept and Self-Esteem, Dr. Gardner recognized that people have different talents and strengths besides being good in school or "book smart." In fact, he identified eight different types of intelligence: visual-spatial—skilled in visualization and art; linguistic-verbal—good with words, language, and writing; logical-mathematical—strong in math and logical problem solving; bodily-kinesthetic—skilled in motor control and physical movement; musical—skilled in rhythm and music; interpersonal—good at understanding others and sociable; intrapersonal—good at understanding ourselves and reflective; and naturalistic—in tune with nature. Although psychologists have argued that these areas may not meet the definitions of "intelligence," they are useful to think about during middle childhood. Between the ages of 6 and 11, children start to express different interests, strengths, and talents. Encouraging a range of activities allows children to explore what they enjoy most and discover if they have particular skills. It is tempting for parents to push children into activities that they themselves like or may have excelled in as children, but it is important to let children choose activities, sports, and hobbies for themselves. Keeping in mind Dr. Gardner's eight types of intelligence is a good way to help your children explore different talents and interests.

One thing that parents need to avoid is not encouraging children to be overly competitive, especially in situations where winning and performance are overly emphasized. At this age, sports and activities should be fun rather than focused on winning or being the best. Parents should say, for example, "I liked watching you play baseball today," or "I liked that new song you were practicing on the violin this evening." Encourage and recognize trying hard, practicing, and doing their best. When activities and sports are no longer fun, or children fear failing and are overly anxious about performing, it is a sign that performance may be emphasized too much by you or others. Parents may need to recalibrate and think about how activities are structured and if coaches or instructors are overly harsh and competitive rather than supportive.

It is important to note that activities do not have to be expensive. There are many free community programs for children through organizations like the YMCA. There are also scholarships and reduced fees available for families who qualify. Summer can be a great time for low-cost weekly camps. You may find that art, theater, and sports camps sponsored by the city parks department and local churches are reasonably priced. Remember to keep a balance between family time and time for outside activities. Kids need free, unstructured time to relax and play with other children, and families need time together for movie and game nights and family meals.

Have Important Conversations

School-age children start to be exposed to influences outside the home on a regular basis, and it is important for parents to be open and willing to have important conversations with children about what they may see or hear about from friends or on television or social media. Unfortunately, there are a lot of tragedies that occur in our world today. The news reports on school shootings, natural disasters, and other tragedies occur all too often, sometimes in our own backyards. When tragic events happen, it is important for parents to talk with their children about these events, to answer their questions honestly, and be a source of accurate information. Parents should also limit children's exposure to media that shows such events because these images can be traumatizing and confusing to children. Parents can comfort children by assuring them that they will do all in their power to keep them safe and explaining that such tragedies, although heartbreaking, are fortunately rare in terms of probabilities.

Parents should also start talking with their children about sex and the facts of life if they have not already. Several resources in the Resources section at the end of this chapter are about how to have these conversations and include books to read with children. It is better for parents to have regular conversations about sexuality as opportunities come up rather than saving it all up for one big talk. If parents do not provide the information to their children, someone else will, and the information and values shared may not be accurate or consistent with your family values.

Another topic that needs to be talked about with children at this age is the effects of discrimination and racism, especially when children experience or see examples of it in their schools, their communities, or the media. Discriminatory policies and racial slurs are unfortunately still common in many settings and can have lasting effects, even when children do not experience them themselves. Rather than taking a "color-blind" approach and ignoring examples of racism and discrimination when they occur, parents should have conversations with their children to bring those situations into the open, talk about why it is hurtful and harmful, and help children develop appropriate ways to respond. Dr. Diane Hughes and her colleagues (2020) have developed guidelines to help parents talk about these difficult topics in ways that are appropriate for school-aged children, particularly when children are members of a minority ethnic, religious, or racial community. Be open to finding ways to help children cope with situations in their schools or communities that cause them distress because of prejudice, discrimination, or racism. More information is provided in the Intentional Parenting for Equity and Justice guidelines listed in Practical Tip 5.2: Conversations About Prejudice, Discrimination, and Race and the Resources section at the end of the chapter.

Practical Tip 5.2: Conversations About Prejudice, Discrimination, and Race

Experts agree that all families should discuss racism and discrimination. A color-blind world is not a reality, and parents need to address this in the home through regular conversations and by encouraging children to have experiences where they interact with different kinds of people and families. All our children attended public schools with students from many different backgrounds when they were growing up. These were intentional decisions on our part because we wanted our children to have friends

> **Practical Tip 5.2: Conversations About Prejudice, Discrimination, and Race (*Continued*)**
>
> from other backgrounds and view the world from multiple perspectives. Along the way, it led to many conversations about history, privilege, and racism and how to handle intolerance, unfairness, or cruelty.
>
> The reality is that many people around the world and in our communities routinely experience prejudice and bullying and fear for their safety. Children benefit when they can talk about these issues. Ignoring the discrimination and injustice that continues to exist in our society is not a helpful strategy for promoting kind and caring behavior in children. Some guiding principles that can help you talk (and listen) to your children about prejudice and discrimination include
>
> - reflecting on your beliefs and how they may impact your thinking and behavior;
> - exposing children to diversity in a variety of settings through school, activities, books, movies, or volunteering and talking about these experiences together;
> - deliberately discussing racism and instances of racial injustice and inequality—when something happens that gains attention in the media, talk about it with your children and ask them what they think and feel and what could have been done differently; and
> - looking for resources online to help guide your conversations—there are some excellent websites that help parents from all backgrounds help their children understand and respond to the unfair and hateful conditions that exist in the world.

Make Rules Together

Discipline during middle childhood becomes easier than at previous ages because children understand the reasons behind rules and limits and can have conversations about expectations and guidelines. In fact, children at this age are often strict enforcers of rules—don't try changing the rules of Monopoly to accommodate a younger child

153

or shorter game time without being prepared for good reasons why a rule can be changed if everyone agrees! The point is that your child now has an appreciation for why rules can make life better and fairer but hasn't yet developed much flexibility about enforcing a rule once it is made. One way you can make sure that your kids are on board with the rules of your household is to involve them in making and understanding them.

In the Active Parenting program we talked about in Chapter 4, you may remember the importance of distinguishing between discipline (teaching) and punishment. Now that children are a little older, a new aspect of discipline involves having conversations with your children about the reasons for family rules and the consequences for breaking those rules. And it helps when children have input and a voice in the process. The Active Parenting program for middle-age children says that even though children may not always get their way, they always get their say (Popkin, 2014). Parents make the final decisions regarding rules, expectations, and consequences for misbehavior, but children should have the opportunity to share their thoughts and ideas about rules and decisions. Parents should consider children's views and opinions, but on important things, parents should have the last word and make the final decision. (See Resources for more information.)

A good way to discuss rules and expectations is through family meetings. This can be a great time to handle disagreements between family members. Family meetings can occur regularly (monthly or weekly) or when families need to discuss a particular issue. Family meetings work best when everyone is allowed to have a say on the topics discussed, and the meeting ends with a game or fun activity. For example, a parent may call a family meeting about keeping the house clean. A child may call a family meeting if a sibling keeps going into their room and getting into their stuff. The meetings are set for a certain time, and all family members discuss the concern raised and come up with solutions together. Parents may have to take a more active role in decision making and planning if children have difficulty agreeing. And note that some rules are nonnegotiable. Those rules are expectations (wearing a seat belt in the car), while other rules may be more negotiable (how much screen time children are allowed on weekends). Family meetings about rules and ways to handle conflict are also a good time to revisit your family virtues and talk about the importance of the virtues that promote a happy and harmonious home life (Popov et al., 1997).

It is important to note that fights among siblings are a normal part of family life. Jennifer vividly remembers hearing the world-renowned pediatrician T. Berry Brazelton talk about sibling conflict at a child development conference when her children were just at that age when their conflicts seemed to escalate in a moment. She never forgot his advice, and her children learned to work out most of their disagreements with limited adult interference. Many experts agree that parents should encourage siblings to handle their own disagreements, only stepping in when support is truly needed, such as when one child is being repeatedly bullied or is overly aggressive (Brazelton & Sparrow, 2005). Of course, there is more that parents can do to teach children how to resolve disputes, such the importance of sharing, taking turns, and imagining the other person's point of view, which should be ongoing. Many parents have an unrealistic goal that sibling relationships are 100% harmonious. Letting them solve most of their squabbles without interfering gives them the opportunity to learn how to deal with conflict, skills that will last a lifetime. Family meetings can be a good time to address sibling conflict if or when it becomes problematic (see Resources section for more information).

Having good routines minimizes the number of rules you have to make and enforce. Many rules are about routines. Bedtime, mealtime, and homework time can all be part of your regular routine and are no longer argued about—unless it's genuinely time to revisit that rule. Then a family meeting can bring in everyone's views, and the rule and routine can be changed. Routines can also help children meet your expectations as a normal part of daily life. Examples include keeping their rooms neat, setting or clearing the table after dinner, and putting dirty clothes in the hamper. When conflicts occur around these basic expectations, it is helpful to decide on and post rules on a family bulletin board or the refrigerator where they can be seen. This might include items such as homework needs to be done before screen time, no snacks allowed an hour before dinner, television programs need to be approved by parents before watching them, and toys or games must be put away after playing. Taking away screen time for misbehavior usually works well, but whenever possible, use natural and logical consequences. For example, if your child keeps forgetting her lunch, one day, she may have to go without lunch rather than having you bring it to her (natural consequence). If your children keep fighting over the iPad, it is taken away for the afternoon (logical consequence).

When Jennifer's son Zack was in second grade, he got a new Gameboy, a handheld video game, for his birthday. Jennifer knew he was playing it a lot but did not realize how much until the teacher told her one day when she dropped him off at school that he had not turned in his homework all week. That evening, Jennifer told him about his teacher's report and that the Gameboy was now only a weekend activity. He surprised her by saying, with obvious relief, "Thanks, Mom. I knew it was out of control." He was grateful that she had helped him control his behavior because he wasn't yet able to do that for himself. This is often the case with video games and other screen-based activities. We need to set limits because children are still developing the self-regulation abilities needed to put those limits in place on their own. Limiting screen time is particularly difficult for children. Millions of dollars are poured into researching how to keep all of us—kids and adults—watching or playing just a little bit longer! We recommend having screen time as part of free time, after homework and other chores are done, or only on weekends if you are not there to monitor it.

This is also a good time to start having conversations about internet content and safety. It is good to have clear rules about online content that kids can view, and parents should monitor and use parental controls when available. More important, parents need to have conversations with children about the dangers of online content. Children need to understand why there are limits and how family values and virtues impact internet rules. Parents will not always be there to monitor screens and online content, so talk with children about what to do if they are at a friend's house and start looking at something that is not allowed at home. The average age that children first see pornography online is 12, according to a survey by Common Sense Media, but 15% reported seeing pornography at age 10 or younger ("Teens and Pornography," 2023). Children need to know how to react when they are exposed to sites that are inappropriate, upsetting, and potentially damaging to them. Internet safety is important, and at the end of this chapter, we provide some helpful resources.

This is a good age for children to start learning about money and get an allowance, even if it is small. Amanda and her economist husband taught their children early about managing money using the three-jar strategy: one jar for saving, one for spending, and one for giving. Many parents like to tie their children's allowance to their chores. We have found that to be difficult. For example, how often do they have to forget a chore to lose all or part of that week's allowance? This can become an accounting nightmare. We think it is better to have a basic allowance that children always get. This way, they can count on it and learn to save up for special things they want to do or have. They should also have basic chores that are part of their routine. Chores are expectations so that children learn how to contribute to the household—not because they get paid but because they are part of the family, and all family members contribute their time and energy to keeping the home clean and free of clutter. We saw in Chapter 4 that even younger children enjoy doing grown-up chores around the house and appreciate being responsible. As children get older, they can handle more responsible and regular chores. Special chores can be rewarded with special incentives, just like adults getting overtime or bonus pay for extra work.

Enjoy Family Time

One of the most wonderful aspects of middle childhood is that children still enjoy spending time with their parents. In a few years, when they become teenagers, they will want to spend more time with their friends, so take advantage of this stage and enjoy your kids. Movie nights, family outings, road trips, and game nights can be fun for everyone. When planning a family night or activity, involve your kids and get their ideas about things to do. You can take turns choosing movies or games, making snacks, or planning special meals or outings. It is a good idea to have a regular day of the week for family nights and invite grandparents or cousins to come regularly if they live nearby.

Reading to your children is still important and can be a great way to wind down before bed or relax after school or chores. Children enjoy hearing parents read more challenging children's books than they are able to read yet. Audiobooks are fun on long commutes or car trips. Games are also a good way for children to practice reading and math. Games such as Scrabble, Monopoly, Uno, and others help children learn rules and strategies and can help build memory and math skills. Partner games such as Spades and group games such as Pictionary are also fun for kids and parents to play together. Relationships thrive when we make time for each other and express our enjoyment of being together. Our lives are often so hectic in today's world that playing seems like an afterthought.

But the time that parents spend at play and having fun with their children and each other is time well spent.

PARENTING CHILDREN WHO HAVE A HISTORY OF ACEs

Families may encounter some specific challenges during middle childhood if their children have already had ACEs. Many children this age have already had or are currently coping with adversity. We share in this book some of the most common situations and encourage you to consider the strategies for coping with them even if this has not occurred in your family. The underlying principles are similar even when specific actions are unique to the situation. These principles include (a) making sure your relationship with your child is strong and sure—they should never doubt your love and acceptance no matter what has happened; (b) making communication a high priority in your relationship—be an open, nonjudgmental, and safe place for your children to share their thoughts, worries, and fears; and (c) providing as many protective and compensatory experiences (PACEs) as you can as part of your daily life and other routines—the accumulation of positive experiences can protect children from and compensate for the harmful effects of adversity and stress.

Divorce

One of the most common ACEs children this age encounter is divorce. One out of four 6- to 12-year-olds will experience their parents' divorce. Divorce is almost always experienced as traumatic by children—that is why it is one of the 10 ACEs. But there are many things that parents can do to lessen the emotional trauma experienced by children whose parents are separating or divorcing. First, recognize that divorce is typically disruptive for children, even when parents do their best to remain on good terms. Children will have negative feelings and lots of questions about why and what will happen to them. Answer their questions as honestly as you can without blaming either parent or sharing information not appropriate for their age and level of understanding. Let them know they are going to be okay. Help them label their feelings and accept them. Reassure them that it is not their fault—almost all children at this age will believe that it was their fault, that if they had behaved better or been different, it wouldn't have happened.

Second, keep the adult conflict away from the child. Don't fight or argue in front of or within earshot of the child. Be polite during pick-up and drop-off times with the other parent. Try to be positive and supportive of the time your child spends with the other parent (except in cases where child abuse was an issue), and don't say negative or derogatory things about them. The more children are exposed to conflict between parents, the more psychological difficulties they will have.

Third, keep routines as consistent as possible. Keep children involved in taking responsibility for their actions and duties. "Catch them" doing good regarding rules and responsibilities—being positive works better than criticizing. When custody is being shared, communicate with the other parent—through a counselor or mediator if it isn't possible to talk with them directly—to discuss living arrangements, rules, and discipline so that you are as consistent as possible in both households. Share important medical and school information with the other parent.

Fourth, let other adults, family members, friends, the pediatrician, and others know about changes in the family so that they are aware and can watch for any signs that your child is having trouble coping. If your child is overwhelmed by the divorce, ask your doctor or school counselor for recommendations for a therapist or counselor. Connect with other families who have gone through similar experiences and are coping well. It is helpful for children to realize they are not alone. Finally, take care of yourself. Find healthy ways to cope with the stress of divorce, such as exercising, getting enough sleep, eating well, keeping a journal, finding a support group, or getting counseling. Recognize that it takes 1 to 2 years before life feels "normal" again. Let go of "what-if" thinking or blaming yourself, your spouse, or others. Give yourself time to recover and recognize the benefits that can come from the change in your life. Good things can and do come from painful experiences. There are many resources available to parents to support children through divorce, including co-parenting apps for scheduling, communicating, tracking expenses, and updating important documents, school records, and medical notes. There are websites and other resources listed at the end of the chapter.

Early Onset of Puberty

Some studies find that children who experience high levels of conflict and family dysfunction are more likely to start puberty early (Hayward et al., 1997). In the United States, puberty usually begins between 8 and 13 years of age for girls and between 9 and 14 years for boys. Puberty plays an important role in development. The hormonal changes during puberty change the body from that of a child to that of an adult. This can be a scary time for kids. The changes in the brain enable more sophisticated thinking skills and a growing development of personal and sexual identity. Many of these changes take years to develop and will be covered in subsequent chapters, but a few points are important in parenting children 6 to 11.

The average age of puberty, particularly in girls, has been decreasing worldwide during the past 40 years. Scientists suspect that changes in nutrition, weight, chemical exposures, and stress may all play a role in the earlier onset of puberty, especially in girls. Sexual abuse is also associated with early onset of puberty in girls. This can be a problem for girls because early puberty is a risk factor for later problems, including depression and risky behaviors such as substance use and early sexual behavior. One of the reasons may be that girls who enter puberty early attract more attention from older adolescents and adults than their peers. For example, a 12-year-old girl whose periods started at 9 may look more like a 15-year-old who started her period at 12. Parents can help their early developing daughters cope with inappropriate attention from older boys and men by limiting who their children can spend time with alone or in groups. They can help them cope with the stress that may arise from being out-of-step physically with their peers by listening to them and helping them develop emotion regulation and coping skills. Emotions are sometimes unpredictable as puberty changes hormone levels, and parents can help children recognize that this is normal and learn how to respond without being alarmed.

Letting your kids know that the physical and psychological changes that occur with puberty are normal helps them be prepared whenever it occurs. One day in the car driving to meet some friends for lunch, Jennifer's 11-year-old daughter Amy asked if she was too young to be going through puberty. Jennifer told her that she wasn't too young to start noticing some changes. Amy replied, "That's good because I feel like crying right now for no reason." That opened an opportunity to talk about how our bodies affect our thoughts and feelings and how the reverse is also true. When parents react calmly and supportively, their kids learn to accept these changes as part of growing up. When children's bodies start to show signs of pubertal development, parents need to reassure them that this is a normal process and be on the lookout for signs of body image problems. Both boys and girls can become obsessed with and unhappy with their physical features as they begin to change. Limiting the amount of exposure to media that promote unrealistic images of either male or female body types is helpful. Watching programs together and commenting about the variety of styles, sizes, shapes, and colors in which beauty can be seen is one way to help children be more accepting of themselves as they become more aware of cultural standards (Harter, 2015).

PACEs in Middle Childhood

As we saw in earlier chapters, PACEs are lifelong methods for ensuring a healthy, resilient, and joyful life as an individual and a family. They provide the structure and routines that support good physical and mental health through relationships and actions. One of the most important ways parents can help their 6- to 11-year-olds develop the qualities that make for resilience is by helping them develop the PACEs they will carry into adolescence and adulthood.

As children go through their elementary and middle-school years, they have opportunities to play different games and sports, join clubs and youth groups, learn artistic and creative skills (music, drama, art, dance), and volunteer to help others. Although it is never completely too late to learn a new skill, learning physical and artistic skills during this age is more likely to lead to success than trying to learn them later in life. Jennifer can't count the number of times she has heard someone say how much they wish they had learned to play the piano when they were young. And every time she says a silent thank you to her parents for making it possible for her to pursue this interest.

Children have little control over their schedules at this age, so parents often have to make real efforts to make time to get children to lessons, practice and sporting events, and other children's houses to play. The first time Jennifer and Amanda presented the 10 PACEs to a roomful of mental health professionals at a conference, one of the questions from the audience was whether they had a refrigerator magnet with the PACEs listed on it. When asked why they wanted one, the respondent said, "I've been trying to do these things for my children, but I hadn't really known why or if they were important—it just felt like the right thing to do. On the days it feels a bit overwhelming, it would be great to see this list on the fridge."

With that in mind, we emphasize that parents must find a balance between taking care of themselves and making sure their children have the PACEs in their lives that will help them be healthy and resilient. One strategy is to carry out the PACEs that support everyone in the family first, such as keeping the house clean and uncluttered, having healthy meals and bedtime routines, and doing active and fun leisure activities together. Make sure that your relationships with each other are supportive and positive by listening and being kind and respectful to each other, agreeing on consequences to help everyone remember the rules, and using family meetings to recalibrate when needed. Then, add special PACEs that support individual children's interests, hobbies, and sports. We know it is often challenging to keep all these balls in the air as you juggle many responsibilities. But the time and effort you put into creating strong relationships and healthy habits will pay off as children learn what to expect, feel supported, and so engage in less disruptive bids for attention, and begin to take pride in being responsible and doing their part in the family. The phrase often repeated about parenting is that "the days are long, and the years are short." In the blink of an eye, you may find yourself in your grown son's home watching his 4- and 6-year-olds proudly showing their grandma how they can empty the dishwasher!

KEY TAKEAWAYS

There is a lot to think about in middle childhood, and next, we highlight some of the most important things to take away from this chapter.

- Recognize the coping patterns that come from your past experiences. Begin to think about how and why these coping strategies developed and which ones are helpful and harmful for you to keep using.
- Encourage your child to try a number of different activities, sports, art, or academic clubs. Be sure to be balanced and not overcommitted. One or two activities at a time are plenty! Let your child choose what they want to focus on and help them find ways to succeed.
- Set limits and make rules together. Let children have a say in the rules, but be the adult and make sure there are clear boundaries in your home. Have family meetings when conflicts arise or changes need to be made.
- Make time for conversations. Children are beginning to have a broader understanding of the world, and parents can be a major influence on their thinking. Talk about internet safety, school and friends, racism and discrimination, and what your child enjoys and why. This is a great time to get to know your children's developing interests, concerns, and unique personalities better. It sets the stage for more in-depth conversations and experiences during adolescence, such as dating, engaging in risky behavior, and setting future goals.
- Have fun together. This is a great time to play board games, attend events together, and support your children's activities and performances. Children enjoy spending time with parents at this age, so take advantage of that and have fun.
- Check in. This is also when many children start to develop mental health problems. If your child is experiencing bullying, let them know they can talk to you. Be ready to intervene and get help, if necessary, by talking with the school, your pediatrician, or friends and family who have experienced this. If your child is going through early puberty, check in and be

sure they are doing okay and understand what is happening in their bodies. If you are getting a divorce, talk with your child openly, and do not hesitate to get help if needed. Internalizing behaviors (anxiety, depression) and externalizing behaviors (aggression, bullying) may become problematic, and getting professional help never hurts.

ACTIVITY: YOU ARE HERE

Parenting is a long journey; it is important to check in and think about where you are and how to make the trip better. Take a few minutes to think about where you are now and answer the following questions.

- What am I doing well as a parent? What do I like most about my child at this age? What do I enjoy most about parenting?
- Where are you in terms of setting limits and granting independence? Do you have clear rules that your child has a say in? Do you encourage your child to engage in a number of activities that they are interested in? Take a few minutes to write down your ideas on where you are with this balancing act and some things you might do differently.
- What PACEs do you currently have? Are there PACEs you need to develop and foster in yourself? If so, which ones? What PACEs are in your children's lives and routines? Are there new or different PACEs that would be good to have? What is your plan for adding them?

ACTIVITY: FINDING YOUR CHAACEs

Many of the coping strategies we used as children experiencing trauma or adversity become habits or ways of thinking and feeling without our being aware of them. For each of the following items, pause and reflect on how you reacted to stressful experiences as a child. In the next chapter, we identify and choose healthy responses to stress to use as adults.

As a child (6–18), when bad things happened to me or others in my home, I often (*circle all that apply*)

- pretended that nothing bad had really happened.
- denied having negative thoughts or feelings.
- refused to believe it had happened.
- avoided being around other people.
- made sure no one knew about the situation.
- took my negative feelings (anger, fear, frustration) out on others.
- fought back verbally or physically.
- distracted myself with video games, TV, food, sleep, drugs, or alcohol.
- was preoccupied with physical aches and pains.
- came up with possible solutions to the problem.
- talked with someone who could help, such as a relative, teacher, counselor, or police officer.
- asked someone I respected for advice and followed it.
- blamed myself for the situation.
- avoided my home and those within it who caused the problem(s).
- worried about what to do.
- told myself it wasn't really happening to me.
- did things to reduce the stress I felt (was physically active, practiced breathing exercises).
- believed that something good would come out of the situation.
- changed something about myself so that I could deal with the situation better.
- tried to make things better by having a plan and following it.

- accepted sympathy and understanding from someone.
- criticized or lectured myself.
- hoped or prayed that a miracle would happen.
- daydreamed or imagined a better time or place than the one I was in.
- had specific fantasies (perfect revenge, finding lots of money) that made me feel better.
- focused on schoolwork, sports, creative interests, or other activities.
- tried to make everything okay by acting more like a parent (caring for younger siblings, doing housework).
- blamed myself for not knowing what to do.
- asked for advice from a school or other counselor and did what they recommended.
- talked with others who had gone through similar situations.

What else helped me survive ACEs or other types of hardship as a child? How were these strategies helpful at the time? What are the downsides of using them?

RESOURCES

Sibling Conflict

Christ, J., & Verdick, E. (2010). *Siblings: You're stuck with each other, so stick together.* Free Spirit Publishing.

Lacovar, J. (2022). *Brothers and sisters: The book for siblings who don't get along.* Puppy Dog Tails & Ice Cream.

Puberty and Sexuality

Mayle, P. (2000). *"What's happening to me?" An illustrated guide to puberty.* Lyle Stuart.

Mayle, P. (2022). *"Where did I come from?" The facts of life without any nonsense and with illustrations* (50th ann. ed.). Citadel.

Schaefer, V. (2012). *The care and keeping of you: The body book for younger girls* (Rev. ed.). American Girls.

Internet Safety

Kids Health online safety: https://kidshealth.org/en/parents/net-safety.html

Common Sense Media media reviews: https://www.commonsensemedia.org/

Internet Matters online safety: https://www.internetmatters.org/

National Society for the Prevention of Cruelty to Children online safety: https://www.nspcc.org.uk/keeping-children-safe/online-safety/talking-child-online-safety/

Discrimination and Racism

Program for Early Parent Support: https://www.peps.org/ParentResources/by-topic/anti-racist-resources-parents

Resilience: https://www.apa.org/res/parent-resources

Ummeh, U. (2020). *How to teach your children about racism*. Teen Alive.

Divorce

American Academy of Pediatrics: https://publications.aap.org/patiented/article-abstract/doi/10.1542/peo_document032/79950/Separation-and-Divorce-Keeping-Your-Children-First?redirectedFrom=fulltext

American Psychological Association: https://www.apa.org/topics/divorce-child-custody/healthy

https://www.helpguide.org/articles/parenting-family/children-and-divorce.htm

https://www.parents.com/parenting/best-co-parenting-apps/

CHAPTER 6

TWEENS AND YOUNG TEENS: BALANCING BOUNDARIES AND AUTONOMY

When it was time for Jennifer's daughter Amy to go from elementary to middle school, she decided she wanted to apply to one of the most rigorous and exclusive private schools in Houston. Amy explained that going to this school would help her get into a great college. Jennifer had some reservations—not about the academics but whether Amy would like it. As an expensive college preparatory school, its student body was different from Amy's public elementary school. However, they decided to try it. Amy took the entrance exams and was accepted along with two of her friends, and everything was off to a great start. Amy jumped right in, making new friends, and Jennifer was delighted with the academics. A few months later, however, some of Amy's sparkle had dimmed. One day after school, Amy confessed that she wanted to go back to public school. Jennifer asked her what was wrong. The work wasn't too hard. She loved her teachers. She was making friends. Amy struggled to find the words to describe how she didn't feel like she belonged there, like there was only a narrow definition of a successful student there. Finally, she blurted out, "It's like their auras are a different color than mine!" And she hastened to add, "I can't really see auras, of course, but if I could, they would be a different color." Jennifer got the message.

This wasn't the right place for Amy. She finished that semester and then went back to public school.

In Texas, we worry about things like ice storms. They are rare but can be devastating. Everything shuts down, schools close, pipes burst. When Amanda was 14, she was at her friend's house with a group of friends when they got word of an impending ice storm. It was already late and dark, so all the kids decided to just spend the night because of the coming ice. Back then, we didn't have cell phones, so the kids (boys and girls) lined up to use the landline and call their parents to let them know the plans. All the parents agreed it was a good idea to stay put, except for one: Amanda's dad. He said simply, "I'll be there to pick you up in 15 minutes." A little embarrassed but not too surprised, she waited until he arrived in his old Ford F150 pickup truck. She climbed in, and they headed home. Neither of them said much. Amanda was a little angry—all the other parents had said it was okay to stay. Why was her family so protective? Amanda's dad probably thought that the chances of the storm weren't too high and they'd have time before it arrived, so why take the risk and have his daughter stuck somewhere with other kids (girls AND boys)? Moreover, she was only 14, and he didn't know her friend's parents. Better safe than sorry. They drove along the country roads, the temperature dropping, passing only a few cars. When they were almost home, her dad calmly said, "I didn't see any ice on the road." There was not much more to say; he was right, and Amanda was safe at home.

MILE MARKERS

These two stories illustrate two types of considerations and decisions parents must make with and for their tweens and young teens. Children this age are starting to think about who they are and how they fit in the world, and they start wanting to spend more time with friends and less time with family. While this is completely normal, it can be difficult for parents accustomed to having more control over their decisions and actions. Tweens and teens want to be independent, but they still need connection with family and protection as they find their places in the world outside of their families.

Physically, children this age are growing into adolescents, especially girls, who are, on average, about 2 years ahead of boys. Girls usually start their menstrual periods during this time, and boys begin to have nocturnal emissions of semen or "wet dreams." While this is normal, it can be initially embarrassing and awkward for them and their parents. When parents can put aside their discomfort and talk honestly and matter-of-factly about the changes their children are experiencing in their bodies, children feel less self-conscious and are more likely to ask questions and share their concerns. Sleep schedules also change when puberty starts. Tweens and teens have difficulty falling asleep at their usual bedtimes as their biological rhythms shift to about 2 hours later than before puberty. Because teens still need 8 to 10 hours of sleep to be healthy and alert, parents often need to help them get enough sleep. Having rules about putting away screens several hours before bed, avoiding food or drinks with caffeine late in the day, and making a good sleeping environment—for example, a comfy pillow, a cool room, and a warm shower before bed—are good ways to help teens get enough sleep and create good nighttime routines.

There is an upside that occurs with the increased need for autonomy and independence craved by our tweens and teens: It primes them to try new things, meet new people, and enjoy new experiences outside of the family. This helps them start to create broader social connections that will hopefully serve them well as they start to transition to young adulthood. The need for independence can cause conflict in families, however. If it feels to you like this stage has the most conflict between parents and kids, you are right! Research has shown that early adolescence is the most volatile time for parents and teens. They tend to disagree over issues related to autonomy and choice ("It is my room; I don't have to clean it," "I can wear what I want"), and conflicts often arise because of different views on reasons for behavior. Parents see such protests as failures in morality or values (my teen is messy and does not value our home; my teen disrespects my authority), whereas teens see these things as a matter of personal choice and opportunities to exert more control over their lives. (See Table 6.1 for the developmental milestones in tweens and young teens; Berk, 2015.)

Major changes are also happening in the brain during this period (see Zooming In 6.1: Brain Development). There are a few psychological concepts that help explain teenagers' thinking. First, by an average age of 12, children can engage in what psychologists call *formal operational thought.* We've seen that children begin looking for logical, cause–effect relationships in preschool and become more capable of understanding rules, logic, and basic scientific concepts during middle childhood. Now, they become able to think logically about abstract ideas—not just physical objects but ideas, principles, the future, and even their own thinking. A whole new world opens up to them as they begin to reason and have feelings about these abstract concepts. They can grapple with more sophisticated moral issues and be outraged by injustice and inequity.

The second aspect of this change in their cognitive development is a preoccupation with themselves—who they are, who they're becoming, and what their position in their social system is now and likely to be in the future. This focus on themselves, or egocentrism, is a normal part of development, but it can lead to some fallacies in their thinking that parents should be mindful of and help protect them from. The first of these has been called the *personal fable,* the idea that teens think they are special and unique, unlike anyone else

TABLE 6.1. Developmental Milestones in Tweens and Young Teens (Ages 12–15)

Age	Physical	Language	Thinking and learning	Social and emotional
12 to 15-year-olds	• Girls: peak of growth spurt; more body fat than muscle; starts menstruation • Boys: begin growth spurt; first ejaculation; voice may deepen • Sleep schedule may start to shift to going to bed later • May have sexual intercourse (14–15)	• Vocabulary continues to increase • Uses and understands abstract words • May adjust the way they talk in different situations	• Scientific reasoning improves • May become more idealistic and critical • Can do basic algebra • Can work with graphs, fractions, percentages • Can use formulas to solve problems • Understands basic geometry • Develops moral reasoning skills	• Becomes more self-aware • Strives for independence • May be moody • Spends more time with peers • May show sexual interest and preferences • Has peer groups based on similar interests • Peer pressure and conformity may increase

Zooming In 6.1: Brain Development

Brain development occurs rapidly in the tween and early teenage years. Puberty sets in motion a number of biological and neurological changes. As scientists, we now know that brain development continues into adulthood and is not complete until the mid to late 20s. What is interesting is that the reward- and sensation-seeking areas of the brain develop earlier in adolescence than the decision-making areas. This means that teens are primed for having fun, meeting new people, trying new things, and risk-taking behaviors (surprised?) before they have the capacity to weigh potential risks and consequences. The prefrontal cortex (PFC) is the last region of the brain to develop, and the PFC is responsible for impulse control, emotion regulation, planning, decision making, empathy, and moral reasoning. So, parents need to be their adolescents' PFC or frontal lobes, protecting them from risks while also encouraging fun behavior that is safe with appropriate boundaries.

in the world. To some extent, this is true, of course, just as no snowflake is exactly the same. However, this way of thinking can have negative consequences. It can increase the likelihood that they'll do risky things because they feel invincible and that bad things cannot happen to them because they are special. Parents must help teens survive this phase in their thinking by creating boundaries and providing support and guidance.

Another fallacy of thinking during this stage is the *imaginary audience*. This is the belief that everyone is watching and noticing them, and everyone will see that pimple on their nose or notice whether they have new shoes. This way of thinking is now reinforced with social media, with the constant tabulation of numbers of followers, likes, and dislikes providing a relentless reminder of their place in the social world. Today's teens often place too much emphasis on the looks and styles of others as they appear on a variety of social media, not realizing that most of what they see is heavily curated and often wildly inaccurate. Research shows a direct effect between time spent on social media and negative self-esteem, especially for girls. As we discuss later in this chapter, tweens and teens are at risk for mental health problems because many types of psychopathology, such as anxiety and depression, typically emerge during this time. It is important to recognize and seek professional help if you see warning signs that your child is experiencing anxiety, depression, or other disturbance in their physical or mental health. Often, problems are much more easily solved when treated early, but our tendency is to hope that things get better on their own. Talk with your child's doctor or school counselor if you see any of the warning signs described in Practical Tip 6.1: Warning Signs of Anxiety and Depression.

Practical Tip 6.1: Warning Signs of Anxiety and Depression

Sometimes it is difficult for parents to know if their child is going through a normal period of emotional distress or whether it is a more serious problem that requires professional care and treatment. Find a quiet moment to sit down and ask them how they are feeling and if anything is bothering them. Most tweens and teens will respond honestly when asked directly. If they say they want to hurt themselves or not be alive, this should be taken seriously. It is important to seek help if you think your child or teenager is depressed or experiencing anxiety that prevents them from engaging in their normal routines. A pediatrician, school counselor, or licensed mental health professional can help by referring you and your child to someone who can do a complete assessment, diagnose the problem, and recommend the right treatments. The good news is that there are many ways to treat depression, anxiety, and other problems that may surface during early adolescence, especially when diagnosed early (see Centers for Disease Control and Prevention, 2023).

(continues)

> ## Practical Tip 6.1: Warning Signs of Anxiety and Depression (*Continued*)
>
> ### Anxiety Symptoms
>
> - being afraid when away from parents
> - having extreme fear (phobia) about specific things or situations
> - being afraid of school and other places where there are people
> - being worried about the future and bad things happening
> - having repeated experiences of intense fear with physical symptoms such as heart pounding, difficulty breathing, dizziness, shaking, or sweating
> - experiencing physical symptoms such as fatigue, headache, or stomach aches
>
> ### Depression Symptoms
>
> - feeling sad, hopeless, or irritable much of the time
> - losing interest in things they once enjoyed
> - experiencing changes in eating—either eating a lot more or less than usual
> - experiencing changes in sleep—either sleeping a lot more or a lot less
> - experiencing changes in energy—being either tired and sluggish or tense and restless a lot of the time
> - having difficulty paying attention or remembering things
> - feeling worthless, useless, or guilty
> - injuring self or engaging in other self-destructive behavior

BALANCING ACTS WITH TWEENS AND TEENS

During this stage, parents have the exciting and challenging task of loving, guiding, and patiently managing their 12- to 15-year-olds, tweens and young teens who think they are much more grown up than they are. A parents' task is to stand alongside them, providing both the limits and structure they still need, along with opportunities to exercise more independent decision making and responsibility.

Fueled by the changes that puberty is generating in their bodies, brains, thoughts, and emotions, our tweens and teens are ready to take on the world. As discussed earlier, the upside of tweens and teens underestimating risks and overestimating their abilities is that they have the confidence, energy, and motivation to try new things. It has been said that young adolescents are like sports cars with great accelerators and faulty brakes. While not entirely true, it may be helpful for parents to think about being their teens' driving instructors, sitting in the passenger seats of the student driver's car, helping them learn to steer clear of potential dangers, anticipating what may be happening farther down the road, knowing when to slow down, and being ready to apply the brakes themselves in an emergency. It is normal to question who they are becoming. And it can be confusing as their bodies are minds are changing rapidly.

There are primarily two areas where parents need to be aware of the need for balance during this age to encourage autonomy while setting appropriate boundaries. First, they must balance being overly watchful or intrusive at one extreme with trusting too much without monitoring at the other. Second, they must balance being overly strict or punitive in response to tweens and teens stretching the limits of their boundaries versus having too few consequences. Finding the right balance in these ways and supporting their questions in regard to identity will result in confidence in your tween or teen.

Research has shown that children need parents to continue to keep a watchful eye on them as they enter adolescence. As their worlds expand—meeting a wider array of students in middle school, sports, or other afterschool programs—they have a broader exposure to others and the world through books, films, music, and other social media (see Resources). They will encounter people, groups, and cultures with values and experiences different from their own. When parents are involved enough to know what their children's homework is about, who their friends are, and what they are watching on their tablets or other screens, they have opportunities to ask them what they think about what they're seeing and hearing.

We saw in the Mile Markers section that at around 12, children not only develop the ability to think more logically about abstract concepts but they also can have strong feelings about those concepts. They begin to hate cruelty to animals, worry about climate change, and love beauty. You will experience this in concrete ways when they announce that they are now vegetarians because they find the thought of eating some other creature's flesh repulsive and immoral, as both Jennifer's and Amanda's daughters did. It is important to stay involved and connected with how your teen is feeling as well as what they are thinking. By asking questions about what they think about issues in the news, events they've attended, or books they're reading, you can generate conversations that open up opportunities to talk about their joys as well as their fears and concerns. And this builds confidence. Finding the balance between being involved and intrusive will differ for each child—and sometimes by the week with each child, but the important thing is to keep talking and listening with an open mind and an open heart. (See Table 6.2 for balanced parenting with tweens and teens.)

TABLE 6.2. Balanced Parenting With Tweens and Young Teens (Ages 12–15)			
Stage and age	**Developmental challenges**	**Balanced parenting**	**Resilient child outcomes**
Tweens and young teens (12–15)	• Questioning versus confusion	• Establishing boundaries versus encouraging autonomy	• Confidence (I am learning who I am; I believe in myself)

In earlier chapters, we have been consistently clear that *discipline*—from the word meaning "to teach"—is more effective than either rewards or punishment in helping children learn how to behave in expected ways. Using rewards and punishment prevents children from internalizing the reasons for healthy and good habits, especially as they get older. For example, giving children a sticker on a chart when they brush their teeth at night may be appropriate for a 2-year-old, but as children get older, focusing on how fresh and clean their mouth feels and knowing that they won't have cavities to be filled by the dentist helps them develop the internal motivation to brush their teeth even when you're not around to remind them.

Likewise, punishment often sends the wrong message—such as "don't get caught" rather than don't do something that will cause pain or problems for someone else or plague their own consciences and self-evaluations. Communicating clearly about expectations and discussing the consequences for violating the agreed-on rules works much better for helping tweens and teens learn how to be responsible for their behavior. Imagine, for example, 14-year-old Zoe, who just started her last year of middle school and thinks she needs (and deserves) to stay up later to manage her increased homework and extracurricular activities. She presents her parents with a proposal that she should be allowed to stay up until 10:30 on school nights instead of 9:30. She has to be up at 6:30 to catch the bus at 7:30, but she argues she will still get 8 hours of sleep. Her parents think she may need more sleep than that (the American Academy of Sleep Medicine recommends that 13- to 18-year-olds get 8 to 10 hours per day; Paruthi et al., 2016) but agree to try it. They all agree that the first time she oversleeps and misses the bus, they will go back to her 9:30 bedtime. Zoe does fine for the first week, but in the second week she almost misses the bus twice and realizes that she's too tired during the day. When her parents point out that the mornings are becoming hectic and that she comes home in the afternoon irritable and exhausted, they all agree that a flexible 9:30 to 10:00 bedtime will work better for her than 10:30. Because she and her parents were on the same side—all of them wanted what was best for her, and they weren't exactly sure what that was yet—there was no drama or fighting about trying a new bedtime and seeing what worked.

Zooming In 6.2: Moral Development

The research conducted by Harvard psychologist Lawrence Kohlberg in the 1970s helps us better understand how our children and adolescents' moral thought and behavior change as they develop (Kohlberg, 1985). Dr. Kohlberg told stories that posed a moral dilemma and asked both adults and children to decide whether a behavior was right or wrong and their reasons for that decision. After analyzing thousands of responses from all over the world, he concluded that moral reasoning skills are linked to cognitive or thinking skills. As children and youth develop the ability to consider broader points of view and understand principles such as fairness and justice, they begin to make more moral decisions.

Kohlberg believed that moral thought and action develop in six stages. Because they don't yet have the ability to consistently take someone else's point of view, young children tend to make moral choices based solely on themselves to *avoid punishment* (Stage 1) or *gain some reward* or advantage (Stage 2). As school-age children begin to understand the need to *conform to social expectations* (Stage 3) and maintain *law and order* (Stage 4), their focus shifts to valuing the importance of the rules (or laws) themselves. As tweens and teens begin to think about society more broadly, they realize that people can agree on moral principles and use them to develop *social contracts* (Stage 5). In the last stage (Stage 6), moral reasoning is based on *universal ethical principles*, much like the values discussed in previous chapters. Now our moral thought and actions are driven by our desire to do the right thing, such as to balance justice with compassion. Ideally, these ethical principles align with local laws and social norms. But there are many situations in human history where they did not, when individuals felt required to break the law to behave morally, such as the "righteous

Zooming In 6.2: Moral Development (*Continued*)

Gentiles" who risked their own and their families' lives to shelter Jews in Nazi-occupied territories during World War II and the nonviolent Freedom Riders in the U.S. civil rights movement.

This is why we recommend using discipline (teaching) rather than punishment or rewards with children from an early age, explaining why actions are right or wrong and how those actions affect others. As they get older, we demonstrate how rules are social contracts that help people live together harmoniously by letting children have a say in setting family rules—and changing them when conditions change. As they become tweens and teens and begin to think and have feelings about ethical principles in action, we listen to their thoughts and share our own. By having conversations as moral issues arise in everyday life, we help them become individuals who can be counted on to do the right thing—not for gain or to be thought of as good, but because they are good.

Sometimes tweens and teens push the boundaries parents set for them because they truly think they are old enough to handle themselves with more independence and responsibility. In these cases, parents need to talk openly with them about why the boundaries are in place—to protect them from situations they aren't ready to handle with older peers or adults. They often don't realize the dangers of being in situations where they could be pressured to use drugs or alcohol, have sex, or engage in other risky behaviors. Parents need to be clear about the consequences that will be imposed if trust is lost when important rules are broken. Parents can ask for examples of how their teens can demonstrate that they are ready for more autonomy and responsibility. Together, they can look for ways for them to demonstrate their ability to be responsible and gain more independence, perhaps by taking on extra paid jobs around the house or in the neighborhood. When they make mistakes, and they probably will, the intent should be to help them figure out what went wrong and how to avoid a similar situation in the future rather than imposing harsh consequences or punishments.

PARENTING WHEN YOU HAVE ACEs: GROWN-UP COPING STRATEGIES

As your child reaches the tween or teen years, you may recall your own struggles during these years. While these memories may be painful, they also provide you with an opportunity to look at them from the perspective of an adult, understanding elements of the situation that were not obvious to your younger self and putting them in their place. As we've recommended before, if these memories are more upsetting than you can handle on your own, look for someone in your community or online who can provide professional support. We list some suggested referral sources in the Resource section.

One way we can make sure that our childhood trauma does not negatively affect how we parent our children is to continue becoming aware of how we manage stress and negative feelings. In the last chapter, we talked about the importance of recognizing our childhood adaptations to adverse childhood experiences (ChAACEs), the third step in breaking the intergenerational cycle of adversity. As you learned, there are many ways children cope with the stress of ACEs, many of which we may not have been aware we were using. As adults, we acknowledge those coping strategies with neither blame nor praise because they were simply our best efforts to cope using the resources we had. Now that we are adults, we want to be more intentional and conscious about how we cope with stress and adversity.

The grown-up adaptations to ACEs (GrAACEs) activity at the end of the chapter provides some structure for reflecting on and choosing how to cope with stress. We start by identifying our current strategies for coping with stress—our GrAACEs—using the list provided and adding others that may not be present. Then we compare them with our childhood strategies from Chapter 5, noticing any patterns that may have persisted. Now we can make some choices, choices probably not available to us when we were young. First, we recommend that you think about strategies that are still beneficial and serve you well. Then decide whether that strategy might need to be modified or used less. We often find something that works for us and then forget that there are other ways to manage stress or negative feelings. For example, many children who distracted themselves from a troubled homelife by working hard and spending time at school doing homework and other activities continue that pattern, working long hours even though they may now have loving families who would enjoy more of their time and attention.

As we decide which strategies to keep, modify, and discard altogether, we like to use a decluttering technique developed by the Japanese home organization specialist Marie Kondo (2014). When working with a family to reduce the clutter and make their homes calmer, she has them hold each item one by one and notice whether that object brings them joy. There are different kinds of joy—usefulness, beauty, comfort—but finding the little spark of joy is the key to knowing whether an object should share one's living space. We think coping strategies are similar. Joy may not be exactly the right emotion, but when you realize that the strategies we use habitually are essentially part of who we are and how we treat ourselves and others, we think they should bring us peace of mind if not outright joy. As you go through the list of GrAACEs, think about the life you want to live and the skills you want to develop and help your children develop, and choose strategies that bring you closer to those goals.

Stepparenting

Another challenge that may arise during this stage is being a stepparent and forming stepfamilies. Many children experience the remarriage of divorced parents by the age of 11 to 15. Parents with a history of ACEs are more likely to divorce than parents with no ACEs and are more likely to remarry at least once. For their children, this may involve sharing their home with a stepfather or stepmother and perhaps with stepsiblings in a "blended" family. Often these families get along just fine, figuring out how to mesh different habits, routines, and rules, but this usually requires some intentional and careful communication between the new spouses and with their children. No matter how much the new couple may love each other—and are prepared to love each other's children—there are some steps and strategies that will make the process of becoming a new family together happen more easily and peacefully.

First, recognize that relationships take time. In general, it takes both adults and children from 1 to 2 years for any change in the family structure, including divorce, the death of a parent, or a new stepparent, to start to feel normal. It takes time to adjust to change and time to get to know, trust, and love new family members.

Second, relationships form more quickly and positively when family members show kindness and respect to each other. Creating expectations about how children will interact with each other and their stepparents is helpful, but most important is for parents to model kindness and respect one another. When parents interact with each other and their children and stepchildren with kindness and respect rather than with harshness, coldness, or sarcasm, they create a culture where children and stepchildren will feel comfortable.

Third, it is important to recognize that stepparents do not have the authority of a parent, but they do have the authority that comes with being an adult who cares and shares responsibility for the family and its children's well-being. A friend of Jennifer's and one of the first psychologists to study stepfamilies, Dr. James Bray, once told her that he recommended stepparents think of themselves as camp counselors. They are not the parent, but they are adults. They should not abdicate the responsibility that rests with an adult when caring for kids, even when they are not their own. Of course, spouses in a blended family need to talk about rules and boundaries and make adjustments where necessary so that children experience as much consistency as possible. When differences exist between the two blended families, make sure everyone understands the reasons for the differences. For example, in one home, there may be three stepsiblings who all attend the same middle school. In this home, the mother's two children are allowed to ride their bikes to and from school together. When the stepfather's daughter is there 1 night a week, she is not allowed to ride her bike with them because her mother does not want her to ride her bike to and from school. These kinds of differences can easily escalate into conflict but are also easily accommodated through good communication.

This example illustrates another potential pitfall for stepparents: co-parenting. If you were co-parenting before adding a stepparent, you should continue co-parenting after remarriage. Just because a parent adds a stepparent into the mix does not negate or decrease the rights or responsibilities of their former spouse, and it certainly doesn't negate the importance of their relationship with the children. If anything, children need to know that the new stepparent isn't a replacement for their mother or father. Both the parent and the new stepparent should be respectful of that relationship. Finally, as a stepparent of tweens and young teens, find ways to get to know your new stepchildren, encourage their interests, and develop a relationship that will help them grow into adulthood. As children of someone you love, it usually isn't too difficult to find things to love about them and ways to show them kindness and affection, recognizing that you're their bonus parent and not a replacement parent. It isn't always an easy transition, but the resulting relationships can last a lifetime.

PARENTING STRATEGIES FOR BUILDING RESILIENCE

Building on the ideas of balanced parenting and developmental milestones for this age, we think the following are important to know about at this stage of the parenting journey. Although we focus more on what can be challenging during this age, we acknowledge that this can also be a wonderful time for parents and teens as their children are growing into adults.

Risk-Taking Behavior

Believe it or not, most experts agree that some level of risky behavior during adolescence is good, particularly during late adolescence and early adulthood. Teens need to take risks to grow and develop into adults. Otherwise, it is hard to meet new people and make new friends, go to new schools, and try new things such as rock climbing and applying for a first job. Parents need to remember during this stage that brain development is not complete (not until the mid-20s), and they need to protect children from risks, particularly during early adolescence. As we said previously, parents need to be their teens' frontal lobes, the part of the brain that helps them make decisions and delay gratification (refer back to Zooming In 6. 1: Brain Development).

Adolescents go through a similar decision-making process as adults; they just weigh the risks and benefits differently. For example, they are much less concerned about safety than adults (remember the personal fable we talked about in Mile Markers at the beginning of the chapter?) That is why it may be difficult to get your teen to wear their skateboard helmet despite your insistence and nagging.

One thing that parents can do is channel their child's energy and need for risk taking into supervised, legal, and more socially acceptable activities such as sports, downhill skiing, surfing, mountain biking, rock climbing, or other activities available in your area. Another thing parents can do is keep their kids busy by encouraging extracurricular activities, volunteering, and hobbies. Children start to make friends at this age that you may not know, and choosing friends who are engaging in risky behavior is something parents worry about. You cannot control your children's choice of friends as they get older, but you can talk with them about what it means to be a good friend and encourage them to spend time in activities with friends who are a positive influence.

Talking About Sex

Many parents are uncomfortable or uncertain about how to talk with their tweens and teens about sex. The key for most parents is to have many conversations rather than the "big sex talk" that makes both parents and kids feel awkward. It is not too late to start if you have not already had these conversations. When kids start to show that they are aware of sex or curious, you can start a conversation by asking them what they already know or think they know. You may be surprised about what they have heard from friends, media, or sex education at school, and you can tailor your conversation accordingly. You may also be surprised about what they do not know or the misinformation they have ("You cannot get a girl pregnant if you wear a condom"), and you can gently correct them ("Well, it lowers the odds, but it is possible because condoms do break"). You might also have resources or links to websites your child can read or look at online without you being present. You can check back with them to see if they have any questions. Sometimes it is easier for a tween or teen to ask an adult who is not their mom or dad the questions they have about sex or other uncomfortable subjects, but it is always good to talk about what they've heard from others. Most kids like learning about the facts without their parents being too involved in the teaching, so they typically welcome the opportunity to read a book or listen to a podcast. You can always ask them to tell you what they learned so you are sure they understand the information.

Romantic Relationships

As we have discovered, the hormonal changes that occur during this age create changes in children's bodies, brains, and behavior. They become more responsive to the physical attractiveness of others, understand and experience the physical and psychological aspects of sexual arousal, and are more aware of their gender identity. Parents' response to these changes profoundly affects their child's mental health and well-being. When tweens begin showing interest in romantic relationships, parents need to listen as well as talk. It is important to have ongoing conversations about healthy relationships, consent, sexual activity, and the consequences of precocious (before the legal age of consent) or unprotected sexual activity. Be prepared and not surprised when your young teens have questions.

Jennifer remembers being on the phone with her brother one Friday night when one of her daughter's 13-year-old friends slipped her a note: "We're talking about poverty and pregnancy if you'd like to join us." She wasn't sure what had prompted this conversation at a routine sleepover, but Jennifer quickly got off the phone and joined the small group of girls who had questions about sex and thought she might be a good parent to ask. A few years later, her daughter told her she liked girls—"really liked them"—and then there were new conversations to have.

Sexual Orientation

In 2021, a national survey conducted by the Centers for Disease Control and Prevention found that 22.5% of high school students said they were gay, lesbian, or bisexual or that they identified in some other way or were questioning their sexual identity, closely matching the 21% of Gen-Z respondents aged 18 and over who identified as members of the LGBTQ community. Parents play an important role in supporting their children's ability to explore their sexual identity and interests without judgment. Many kids try to suppress their feelings to fit in with the mainstream heterosexual culture they see in the media and around them and may fear upsetting their parents or families. Children and teens who are unable to talk about their feelings are at risk for depression and other mental health issues.

In contrast, having a supportive relationship at home and good relationships with friends help them develop a positive identity. Jennifer asked her daughter Amy, who is now an adult and an artist who teaches printmaking to college students, for her advice for parents of tweens and teens. Her first admonition to parents is not to assume a hetero-centric vision of your child's future or the world. Recognize the variety of sexual orientations that exist, be aware of biases you may have, and try not to share them. Second, make sure that your LGBTQ child knows that you love them and will always love them. Third, reassure them that the world will love them! True, there are still people and communities that may not accept them, but let them know that they will find communities who will love them—not in spite of who they are, but because of who they are. Finally, recognize that it's normal to feel some grief for the identity you assumed your child would have, particularly for trans kids. Find other outlets for your feelings, such as parent support groups, so that you don't burden your child with your feelings (see Practical Tip 6.2: Gender Identity).

Practical Tip 6.2: Gender Identity

As tweens and teens begin to develop their sense of who they are, they may question their sexual orientation and gender identity. It is a topic that many parents are reluctant to bring up, fearing that they will somehow make things worse if they don't say the right thing or handle it well. In fact, the best thing parents can do is be prepared—not necessarily with information, but with an open and caring attitude. Some children are sure from an early age that their physical and mental genders are not aligned. Others gradually realize that they do not feel at home in the gender to which they were assigned. Because society has only recently begun to openly accept more diverse gender identities, many parents did not grow up talking about this.

One of our friends gave us some good advice for parents. Her teen told her several years ago that he feels like a boy and not a girl. Today, her son getting hormone treatment and supportive care at the Center for Gender Diversity at Children's Hospital in Colorado. She recommends that parents seek professional medical care and psychological support to help their child as well as the rest of their family with the process. It allows everyone to know what to expect and to deal with the stress that accompanies change and helps family and friends to be supportive. Our friend also echoed Jennifer's daughter's advice to keep communication lines open.

Exploring one's gender identity is a process just like other aspects of identity development, and parents' support and encouragement are key. Our friend added that it has been helpful to make their home a safe place for her son's friends because some of them do not have parents who are able to accept their journey. The road hasn't been without bumps. They are homeschooling this year because kids at school were often hateful, and homeschooling during the pandemic was much less stressful as a result. Our friend admitted to sometimes grieving over no longer having a daughter but says that the benefits of having a son who is happy and comfortable with himself are worth it. She said, "My child is my child—he's still the same person, but now he's a boy."

It is important to continue talking with your children about internet safety (also see Chapter 5). Before kids get their first phone, we recommend having them write a contract with rules and limits. You may be surprised how thorough and good your children are at coming up with their own rules. At a minimum, you should have rules about when and how phones are to be used (not during family meals, only for calling and keeping up with friends on approved sites) and that they should expect you to monitor their phone activity and contacts. That means that they share their passwords with you. It is a good idea to have a charging station in a shared room, such as the kitchen, where everyone can plug in their phones at night at a set time. It's a good idea to have all screens off for an hour before bedtime. This encourages children to read for school or fun before bed, a great habit to get into.

Being With

In the movie *Little Miss Sunshine* (Dayton & Faris, 2006), the teenage son, Dwayne, wanted to be a jet pilot. If you've seen the movie, you may remember the wacky family and their eventful road trip to the child beauty pageant. On the trip in the family van, Dwayne learns that he is color-blind when his sister asks him to identify color patterns on a test for color-blindness. Color-blind people cannot fly jet planes. When he realizes this, he has a complete meltdown in the van, hitting his head against the van window, and his parents pull over on the side of the road. He gets out of the car and runs down a rocky hill, yelling expletives. He believes his whole life is ruined. Mom tries to talk with him, but he screams at her and wants to be left alone. As the family stands on the side of the road, wondering what to do, little Olive (his sister, Miss Sunshine) walks down to Dwayne and simply sits next to him. She puts her arm around him and her head on his shoulder but says nothing. After a few minutes, Dwayne gets up and walks to the car.

This story illustrates the concept of *being with* that comes from the Circle of Security program (Hoffman et al., 2006). Recall from Chapter 3 the Circle of Security figure that portrays secure attachment, with strong hands representing the parent, the top of the circle representing child exploration, and the bottom of the circle representing returning to the parent when unsure or afraid. Attachment in adolescence comes from these early experiences in childhood but looks a little different. An attached teen may go to a parent for advice, but often, the teen wants to solve problems on their own. The strategy of being with represents the parent walking alongside their child. Simply be present, perhaps giving some comfort (a smile, a hug) and just being available so the teen knows they are not alone. Tweens and teens desperately want to be independent and solve things on their own, so simply being around and available provides the reassurance they need to keep themselves moving forward.

Practical Tip 6.3: Family Meals

One excellent way to be with your child is to have family meals together. It does not always have to be dinner because that can be a challenge with activities and sports. For a while, Amanda's family had regular breakfasts together because of evening soccer practice schedules, and this worked well. There is abundant evidence that children who eat regularly with their families do better in school, have better overall mental health, and have fewer physical health problems such as obesity. Scientists think this occurs for several reasons. First, it is a time to share conversations and learn about daily activities, such as what was fun, what was stressful, what surprised them, and what they are looking forward to. Such conversations strengthen the parent–child relationship and parent involvement in the child's life. Second, parents can make sure teens are eating nutritious foods, with fruits and veggies and not too much sugar or caffeine. Third, it is a time to have conversations about what is going on in the broader

---

Practical Tip 6.3: Family Meals (*Continued*)

world and about moral issues that arise in the media and everyday life (see our ideas on ways to involve tweens and teens in the community in the section on volunteering). This is a good time to talk about topics they may be thinking about but don't always bring up in the hustle and bustle of daily life. While sitting down and eating, you can ask your kids about their thoughts on issues in the news, share your views, and talk about the moral and ethical issues involved (refer back to Zooming In 6.2: Moral Development). Be ready for your teens to disagree with you. This is normal and a good thing! It means they are starting to think about and develop their own moral values and ethical principles. Research has shown that parents' ideas are still important to teenagers—even more important than their friends' ideas. Mealtime conversations about important topics are one way you can continue to influence their thinking and the person they are becoming.

Monitoring

Hundreds of studies have shown that children do better—they engage in less risky and deviant behaviors—when their parents know where they are, who they spend time with, and how they spend their money. Parents can monitor their children in a variety of ways. With cell phones and tracking apps, this is easier than it was in the past. But parents need to let their tweens and teens know they are monitoring their whereabouts. Make this part of the requirement for spending time away from home or having a phone, and it will become second nature. One of the best ways to monitor behavior is for children to tell their parents what they are doing and how they are spending their time and money. Children can spontaneously share this information or share it in response to a parent asking questions during normal conversations. Monitoring becomes even more important and challenging when children start driving or have friends who drive. By this time, it is good to expect family members to share their whereabouts and plans with one another. Parents can also find out information through other parents and adolescents' friends. As mentioned in other chapters, it is important to make friends with other parents and have regular contact with the families that your children spend time with. Then, you can easily check with them when your kids are planning sleepovers, and you can share concerns and help watch out for each other's kids.

Spending time together and having a good relationship with your teen makes monitoring natural and easy. Children are more likely to share things about themselves and their lives when you spend time together one-on-one or during family meals. Plan times to be together and listen when your teen shares. Try to respond in a nonjudgmental way. Another great way to monitor your child is to simply observe. You may be surprised how much you can learn while carpooling—just by staying quiet! Also consider "friending" your tween and their friends on Instagram when they are young rather than waiting. It is more natural then, and teens will get used to their parents seeing their posts and their friends' posts, and it won't feel so intrusive if it is the way things have always been.

Rules and Consequences

In addition to monitoring, it is crucial for parents to have rules and enforce consequences for breaking rules. This sets the stage for later adolescence when it becomes more difficult to enforce rules and closely monitor behavior. At this age, rules regarding homework, screen time, chores, drugs, alcohol, and curfew are all important. Parents want to build good habits and communication patterns, and it is easier to trust your teen when you have established boundaries and communicated that limits exist because you care. Parents can even say, "I trust you, but I don't trust other people on the road," or "We all need routines and habits to stay on track, and this is what we do in our family." Teens may complain about rules, that they are unfair or that they are the only ones whose families have them (remember Amanda's ice storm story?), but when researchers ask teens about rules, they admit that they understand why there are rules and know it is because their parents care for them. As teens get older, kids report that they are glad their parents had rules and that it helped them to do the right thing when other teens were getting into trouble. Teens who do not have rules often feel that their parents don't care about them or are too busy with their own lives to be involved anymore.

As with other ages, create rules and set expectations together, and allow teens to have input. It is a good idea to agree on logical or natural consequences for breaking a rule to avoid arguments in the future and so teens know what to expect: "If you come home past curfew, you won't be able to do things with your friends for a week"; "If you don't get your homework done, and your grades suffer, we will take away your phone [a logical consequence] except for homework until things improve." When it comes to drugs and alcohol, observe your teens' behavior closely. When they come home after being with friends, have them check in with you and give them a hug. If you smell marijuana or alcohol, have a conversation the next day. Ask them what happened and remind them of the rules and consequences ("No going out with friends for 2 weeks"; "We must talk with the parents before you can go to their house"). It is a good practice to let kids know that you will regularly go into their rooms, and if you find drugs or alcohol, there will be consequences. If things escalate, seek help. The earlier kids start drinking alcohol and using illegal drugs, the more likely they will have addiction problems later. There are resources at the end of the chapter that talk about how to handle adolescent drug use and drinking.

PARENTING CHILDREN WHO HAVE A HISTORY OF ACEs

Children who have experienced adversity by the ages of 11 to 15 are old enough to begin to process their experiences. They may begin to compare their experiences with those of their friends and peers and wonder why their lives have had more (or less) trauma than those around them. They may wonder what they could or should have done differently, blaming themselves for their trauma or their reactions to it. The most important response a parent can make when their tweens and young teens express these thoughts and feelings is to listen. Listen with full attention and no judgment. Help them clarify or label their feelings. Reassure them that whatever happened to them was not their fault, no matter what they did or didn't do. Children are not to blame for abuse, neglect, or other adversities that happened. If they express interest in talking with someone who is trained to help them handle their feelings, follow through with getting an appointment and taking them to see a trauma-informed therapist or counselor. Their pediatrician or school counselor should be able to make a referral to an appropriate professional, and there are resources listed at the end of the chapter. The earlier a child is able to talk with someone about their traumatic experiences, the earlier they can begin to recover, recognize and release shame and other negative feelings, and develop positive ways to manage negative thoughts and memories. Most counselors will include the parents in the process, and this is an excellent way for parents to learn and feel more confident in supporting their children's recovery and development following traumatic experiences.

Earlier in this chapter, we discussed GrAACEs, and we provided a list of ChAACEs in Chapter 5. As you now know, these survival strategies often serve a useful function in the short term, helping children manage, cover up, or deny the stress and pain they experienced. However, the same strategies may prevent them from connecting genuinely with others, trusting themselves, or experiencing intimacy as adults with trustworthy partners. As children enter adolescence and begin to look for patterns, find explanations, or search for meaning in their experiences, parents can help them identify both the positive and negative ways they have coped and adapted to childhood trauma. Tweens and teens are not too young to begin to reflect on the coping strategies they use and whether they are of continued value (see the tween and teen ChAACEs activity).

Creating a Story

Research has made clear that keeping traumatic experiences buried and unspoken is not the best route to recovery. While reliving the trauma—complete with physiological responses and emotional memories—is not recommended unless guided by a trained professional, it is helpful to acknowledge that (a) bad things happened, (b) it wasn't your child's fault, (c) you are sorry they have suffered as a result, and (d) sometimes both good and bad things are learned from trauma. For example, adults who have experienced mistreatment may find it more difficult to trust others, but they also may be more empathic to other people's suffering and more likely to become someone who helps others (teacher, nurse, counselor, police officer). When they are open to these conversations, parents can help their children retell their story, in which they see themselves as the surviving hero of the story rather than a victim, get professional help as needed for themselves and their children, and look for ways to find meaning in their experiences.

PACEs for Tweens and Teens

As children become teenagers, they naturally want to have more influence over their daily routines, habits, and activities. While parents want to watch for unhealthy patterns (too much junk food, too little sleep, too little physical activity or study time), this is a good time to support them in adjusting their routines to fit their needs and interests. Continue to encourage and support outside interests such as sports, creative activities, friendships, and volunteering. Also encourage them to take more responsibility for household chores, knowing that in a few years, they will need to know how to do laundry, make a grocery list, stick to a weekly expense budget, or wash the car. You can share how you balance time for fun activities with responsibilities and chores. Boredom is a young adolescent's worst fear and a parent's enemy—kids rarely get into trouble when they are actively engaged in engrossing and challenging activities. Look at the categories of PACEs with your teen (Chapter 2) and update them to match their current interests and goals.

Making sure that tweens and teens have both the supportive relationships and resources outlined in the 10 PACEs ensures that they continue to develop resilience and recover from childhood adversity. As children get older, they may feel embarrassed by displays of physical affection, but they still need to hear that their parents love them unconditionally. Parents may not like certain aspects of their behavior, but children should not worry for a moment that they aren't loved. Particularly when there are changes in the family structure following divorce and remarriage, it is important to maintain stability and consistency through routines, friendships, physical activity, sleep, and healthy food and spending time on interests and hobbies. Tweens and teens may be reluctant to share their thoughts and feelings as readily as they did during earlier years, valuing their privacy and worrying about what others think of them. Helping them maintain their interests more independently will benefit their need for autonomy while also keeping them connected to the positive experiences that build resilience and buffer the effects of adversity.

During this age, having rules and routines is important, as we noted previously. One routine that is especially valuable is having family meals (refer back to Practical Tip 6.2: Gender Identity). This gives families a time to catch up on day-to-day activities, as well as talk about important things going on in the community and broader world, such as challenges for countries facing an influx of refugees fleeing from conflict and war or how to help families in need who have experienced a natural disaster. Many tweens and young teens thrive on volunteering and getting involved in community activities and social causes at this age. They are starting to form their own values and opinions, and a good outlet for channeling this new energy is community involvement and activism. Volunteering at a local food pantry or for an organization that promotes recycling or cares for homeless pets or being involved in groups such as scouts or faith-based organizations can be an important protective factor during these formative years. Many youths benefit from group mission trips where teens volunteer to help communities in need, such as helping clean up after a hurricane or repairing homes in low-income neighborhoods. Such activities give them a different perspective and challenge their way of thinking about the world. And as a bonus, they often gain useful skills such as basic carpentry or home repair.

KEY TAKEAWAYS

As in previous chapters, here we summarize some of the main points to remember from the chapter to help you use the balanced parenting strategies to facilitate resilience in your tween or teen and yourself. As parents, we are much happier when our kids are doing well!

- Think about and choose the coping strategies you want to continue using as an adult. Talk with your child about their coping strategies, too (see Activities).

- Be sure you are monitoring your child's behavior. Do you know where they are, who they are spending time with, and how they are spending their money? Remember that tweens and teens who have parents who monitor their behavior are less likely to get into trouble or have friends who do.
- Are you talking enough with your child? Make time to talk with them about what they are doing, their activities, and their friends. Show interest and learn about what they like to do and how they like to spend their time. It is also important to have regular conversations about risky behavior such as drug and alcohol use, surfing the internet, sex, and other concerns you may have.
- Is your teen getting adequate sleep? Sleep plays a major role in our physical and mental health, and many tweens and teens today do not get enough sleep. This affects their schoolwork, how they feel, and their mental health. At this age, kids need about 9 hours of sleep at night; the time that they naturally fall asleep is getting later, so be sure to check in, have a plan, and help them plan their evenings so that sleep isn't lost.
- These are the years that many mental health problems begin to emerge, such as anxiety, depression, and substance use. Check in with your child. If they seem down all the time, like they're not enjoying their usual activities, or overly anxious about school, and it is impacting their schoolwork, have conversations with them and get professional help. If your child is starting to experiment with drugs and alcohol, have conversations and consider getting help. Experimenting with drugs and alcohol is normal during middle and late adolescence, but early use by tweens and young teens is a risk factor for later problems.
- As with all ages, there are many things to celebrate during this stage! Despite the risks we've discussed, enjoy how your child is growing into an adult. They are becoming an individual with

their own thoughts and ideas. There are lots of exciting things ahead (driving is one of them!), and it is important to delight in the activities and interests of your child while you can.

ACTIVITIES: YOU ARE HERE

Take a minute to think about where you are with balancing the competing demands of boundaries and autonomy. Do you have sufficient rules and boundaries to protect your child? Is your child involved in making decisions about rules and consequences? Are you having regular conversations with your child about safety and risky behavior, and are you asking their opinions and ideas regarding risk and protection? In general, ask yourself the following:

What am I doing well as a parent? What do I like most about my tween or teen? What do I enjoy most about parenting my child at this age?

What PACEs do I currently have? Are there PACEs that I need to develop and foster? If so, which ones? What is my plan for building those PACEs for my child?

Childhood Adaptations to ACEs (ChAACEs) for Tweens and Teens

As we saw in the Mile Markers section, most children begin to think differently at around 11 or 12. They begin to think about and have feelings about such abstract concepts as injustice and ethics and start to think about possibilities, the future, and even their own thinking. And, of course, they think about themselves and their place in the world (more on this in the coming chapter). This is an opportune time for them to think about the coping strategies they may have used in the past. Most early adolescents are capable of reflecting on which strategies they want to use now and in the future and which childhood strategies are no longer of value to them.

Just as in Chapter 5, we invite you to show the shortened list of Childhood Adaptions to ACEs to your tween or teen so they can consider their coping strategies and these questions on their own. They may find this useful even if they haven't experienced ACEs. Offer to talk about ones they would like to keep, drop, or add. If they ask, be willing to talk about the ChAACEs that you once used to deal with adversity. Make a point of not being judgmental—they all serve a purpose in our childhoods, no matter how unhelpful they may be when used later in life in other circumstances. Then when you notice your teen using a positive coping strategy and it's appropriate to remark on it, let them know you see them coping in healthy ways. Learning good coping strategies is a lifelong process, and we can all use all the support we can get from those around us!

Childhood Adaptations to Adversity for Your Tween or Teen

In the past, when bad things happened to me or others in my home, I often (*circle all that apply*)

- pretended that nothing bad had really happened.
- made sure no one knew about the situation.
- fought with others verbally or physically.
- distracted myself with video games, TV, food, sleep, drugs, or alcohol.
- was preoccupied with physical aches and pains.
- talked with someone who could help, such as a relative, teacher, counselor, or police officer.
- blamed myself for the situation.
- avoided my home and those within it who caused the problem(s).

- did things to reduce the stress I felt (was physically active, practiced breathing exercises).
- believed that something good would come out of the situation.
- daydreamed or imagined a better time or place than the one I was in.
- focused on schoolwork, sports, creative interests, or other activities.

Questions for reflection:

- What else helped me survive adversity or other stressful situations when I was younger?
- How were these strategies helpful at the time?
- What are the downsides of them?
- What strategies would I like to let go of?
- What coping strategies would I like to use more in the future?

Choose Your GrAACEs

In Chapter 5, you looked at the coping strategies you may have developed in response to stress and adversity as a child or adolescent. In this chapter, we invite you to think about the strategies you currently use to deal with stressful or difficult situations. Circle those you sometimes use and reflect on the strategies you could use to be more resilient.

As an adult, when bad things happen to me, I sometimes (*circle all that apply*)

- pretend that it's not really so bad.
- deny having negative thoughts or feelings.
- refuse to believe it happened.

- avoid being around other people.
- make sure no one knows about the situation.
- take my negative feelings (anger, fear, frustration) out on others.
- fight back verbally or physically.
- distract myself with video games, TV, food, sleep, drugs, or alcohol.
- am preoccupied with physical aches and pains.
- come up with possible solutions to the problem.
- talk with someone who can help, such as a relative, clergy, or police.
- ask someone I respect for advice and follow it.
- blame myself for the situation.
- avoid being with those who caused the problem(s).
- worry about what to do.
- tell myself it wasn't really happening to me.
- do something healthy to reduce stress (be physically active, practice breathing exercises).
- concentrate on finding something good that could come out of the situation.
- change something about myself so that I can deal with the situation better.
- try to make things better by having a plan and following it.
- accept sympathy and understanding from someone.
- criticize or lecture myself.
- hope or pray that a miracle will happen.
- daydream or imagine a better time or place than the one I am in.
- have specific fantasies (getting the perfect revenge) that make me feel better.
- focus on work, sports, creative interests, or other activities.
- try to make things better by being extra responsible and caring for others around me.

- blame myself for not knowing what to do.
- get professional help and follow their recommendations.
- talk with others who have gone through similar situations.

Questions for reflection

- How else do I cope with adversity now?
- What strategies would I like to let go of?
- What coping strategies would I like to use more?

RESOURCES

Parenting Tweens and Teens

Steinberg, L. (2011). *You and your adolescent: The essential guide for ages 10–25*. Simon & Schuster.

Steinberg, L. (2014). *Age of opportunity: Lessons from the new science of adolescence*. Eamon/Dolan.

Active Parenting of Teens: https://activeparenting.com/product/active-parenting-of-teens/

Internet Safety

TeensHealth online safety: https://kidshealth.org/en/teens/internet-safety.html

U.S. Department of Justice: https://www.justice.gov/coronavirus/keeping-children-safe-online

Preventing Problem Drug Use and Mental Health Problems

Substance Abuse and Mental Health Services Administration: https://www.samhsa.gov/find-help/prevention

American Psychological Association: https://www.apa.org/topics/parenting/helping-kids

American Psychological Association crisis hotlines and resources: https://www.apa.org/topics/crisis-hotlines

Moral Development

Coles, R. (1998). *The moral intelligence of children: How to raise a moral child*. Plume.

Sexuality, Sexual Orientation, and Gender Identity

Centers for Disease Control and Prevention LGBTQ+ youth resources: https://www.cdc.gov/lgbthealth/youth-resources.htm#family

Decluttering Your Home and Your Life

Kondo, M. (2014). *The life-changing magic of tidying up: The Japanese art of decluttering and organizing*. Ten Speed Press.

Resources for Tweens and Teens

Bowe, F. (2022). *Life skills for tweens: Everything a pre-teen should know to be a brilliant teenager*. Bemberton.

Moss, W., & Moses, D. (2015). *The tween book: A growing-up guide for the changing you*. Magination Press.

CHAPTER 7

OLDER TEENS AND YOUNG ADULTS: BALANCING LETTING GO AND STAYING INVOLVED

The message came through Facebook Messenger. A friend of Jennifer's son Zack was reaching out to her because she had just talked to him by phone and was worried. Zack was working part-time and living in a small set of rooms in an art gallery, figuring out what he wanted to do in the next stage of his life. But according to his friend, he now had no money and no food until the end of the month. Mama Jennifer swung into action. She called Zack, who told her he was okay, but she wasn't convinced. She called her husband, Zack's stepfather, who was out of town, and he agreed that she should fly down and drive back with Zack to Tulsa in his car. She transferred some money from her bank account to his so he wouldn't starve, packed a bag, and got a flight to Houston. When she got to Houston, Zack seemed unusually calm for someone on the brink of starvation, but he had packed all his things into his car as she had asked. They made the 8-hour drive back to Tulsa and spent the next several days talking. Jennifer discovered that Zack did have a plan for the future; he just hadn't laid it out until then. She realized she needed to trust him to find his own way. A few days later, he packed his things back into the car and drove back to his life in Houston. Zack hadn't really needed to be rescued, but Jennifer was still glad she made the trip.

Zack's version of the story: It was the summer of 2009 in Houston, Texas. I was 20 years old, and I had recently quit an extremely demanding and stressful job. In fact, I had been working 60+ hours a week with multiple jobs since I was 17. I decided it was time for a break. I had a friend who owned an art gallery and needed someone to live there to watch over the place and let artists in at all hours of the night to drop off and pick up their work. The landlord owned several properties around town, and he would occasionally pay me to do odd jobs such as siding, roofing, and insulation. I made, at most, $100 per week, but there was always food and beer left over from art shows. I slept on an air mattress and spent most of my days outside in the sun, working with my hands and learning maintenance and construction trades. Most of my nights were spent socializing at parties at the art gallery. Looking back, it was truly the best summer of my life. For the first time, I was without responsibility and free to explore who I was. I suppose it was my budget version of "back-packing across Europe." I was having a great time right up until my mother called and told me that someone had called her and told her that I was homeless, starving, and drinking every day, which, technically, was true: I would go days with just leftover cheese cubes, crackers, and beer as my only calories, spending what little money I had on ice to keep the kegs cold. For a 20-year-old, however, this was an ideal living situation, and I was the envy of a lot of my friends who were still living at home, bound by parental supervision. My mother, however, did not agree. I spent a week in Tulsa, getting more and more depressed. I finally decided that I didn't care what my mom thought; I had confidence in myself and my future, and I knew what I was doing with my life.

I think I left on mixed terms. I remember being angry that my mother and stepfather did not seem to trust me to make my own decisions with my life. When I got back to Houston, however, things were not the same. I no longer wanted to sleep on an air mattress in an art gallery and eat stale cheese and crackers. I soon found a real job and, eventually, an apartment, and within 6 months of returning from Oklahoma, I was enrolled in community college. Now, I am a summa cum laude graduate of the University of Houston Honors College, earning a six-figure income, with my own family and multiple beds in rooms of my own to sleep on. I still look back on that summer as the best summer of my life, but sometimes I wonder if my mom had not shown up and ruined my good time, whether I would still be doing odd jobs, drinking warm beer, and sleeping on the floor. I would like to think that I would have eventually figured it out, but maybe it would have taken me a little longer.

Jennifer and Zack clearly had different perspectives then and different memories now of this event, but they both agree that it worked out for the best. Their stories beautifully illustrate the main balancing challenge of this age range, letting go while staying involved.

MILE MARKERS

The developmental period of older adolescence and young adulthood is often stressful for families. It is a time of renegotiation—new roles and identities form, and adolescents are becoming adults. Physically, their bodies can reproduce, and they don't look like children anymore. Mentally, their brains are continuing to develop. Socially, they still need their families, but they also need their friends. Many parents struggle during this time because it is difficult to transition and let go, and it is normal to worry about our children. Amanda remembers Jennifer telling her when her children were entering adolescence that parenting during childhood is physically exhausting, but parenting during adolescence is mentally exhausting. We have both found this to be true. Understanding development and the natural conflicts teens and young adults are going through can be helpful as parents navigate the often-challenging part of this journey.

During the 16- to 18-year age range, some important milestones are typically reached—driving, dating, graduating from high school, and leaving home for college or work. This newfound independence can be challenging for parents but can also be a wonderful time as parents watch their children grow into young adults with their own thoughts, goals, and dreams. Physically, girls mature before boys, and by early adulthood, most adolescents have completed their growth spurt. Thinking continues to become more abstract, and adolescents start to think about their future and what they want to do after school. Many rites of passage occur during this time—registering to vote, obtaining a driver's license, and earning money at a regular or part-time job. Many teens are beginning to feel less self-conscious and more confident. As we discuss later in this chapter, adolescents often actively explore their identity and spend time thinking about who they are, who they want to be, and what it may take to get there. Dating is more common, and relationships outside of the family become more important. Nevertheless, maintaining connection during this time is crucial for resilience.

Zooming In 7.1: Parents and Teens' Brains

Amanda's research lab has been studying how parents influence teenage brain development in a number of studies over the past decade. She and her students have used a variety of methods to see how teens' brains respond to parents in real time. For example, they have looked at how adolescent brains respond to mothers' praise and criticism during discussions about how to resolve parent–teen conflicts and when mothers talk with their teens about something upsetting, such as breaking up with a boyfriend. Her lab uses functional magnetic resonance imaging (a neuroimaging technique) to examine how different areas of the teenage brain respond during these different scenarios.

Zooming In 7.1: Parents and Teens' Brains (*Continued*)

Several findings from this research are relevant to parenting adolescents. First, we can actually see that what parents say affects different areas of their children's brains. For example, adolescents with more symptoms of depression have heightened amygdala responses when they hear criticism from a parent (Aupperle et al., 2016). The amygdala is the region of the brain that responds to threat and triggers emotional responses (the "smoke alarm" part of the brain we talked about previously). Second, we believe that these brain responses affect brain development over time because much of the structural and functional development of the brain is in response to social interactions and context. Third, during adolescence, brain regions involved in emotion regulation and emotion processing are highly active during these conversations, signaling that parents are having an impact not only on adolescent behavior but also on their brain functioning—specifically in relation to emotion regulation.

Interestingly, our studies also show that adolescents influence their parents' brains too. In one study, we had both parents and teens in two MRI scanners at the same talking to each other about a problem. The parents' cortical brain regions, involved in thinking and regulation, were activated when the teens' anterior insula was activated (Ratliff et al., 2021). The anterior insula is considered an emotion hub of the brain; this finding suggests that parents' brains actively work to regulate their response to teens' emotional arousal. So, what parents say to their teens does matter! It affects their brain and development, and kids affect their parents' brains, too.

As we have seen, brain development continues into the mid-20s. The frontal regions of the brain responsible for decision making, moral reasoning, and emotion regulation continue to mature, making it important for parents to still check in and provide support when needed. In fact, young adults' tendency to hold onto the personal fable thinking (described in the previous chapter) may continue to make them feel invincible, as if they can accomplish anything and nothing bad can happen to them. All of this makes it important for parents to stay involved in their kids' lives.

Most young adults have begun to assess more fully their strengths and weaknesses and have identified some possible career goals and pathways to achieve them. But they may also encounter obstacles and find themselves rethinking those goals. Parents can serve as good sounding boards for them as they think through alternatives and sort through their thoughts and feelings about the process. Many young adults begin more serious romantic relationships, if they have not already done so, and learn how relationships work, experiencing both the highs and lows of romantic attachments. This can be a thrilling time of love, loss, heartbreak, and adventure. Sometimes it is difficult for parents to observe this angst and excitement without getting overinvolved at one extreme or wanting to step out of their kids' lives altogether at the other. The key task for parents is learning how to let go while still remaining involved in appropriate and helpful ways. (See Table 7.1 for developmental milestones in older teens and young adults; Berk, 2015.)

BALANCING ACTS DURING ADOLESCENCE AND EARLY ADULTHOOD

The big challenge for parents and kids alike during this stage is to navigate their leaving home with as little drama and as much love and support as possible. A parent's task is to stay connected and supportive while allowing their children to separate and make their own life. As we saw in Jennifer's so-called "rescue mission" with her son Zack, it isn't always easy to know when they need your help and when they just need time to figure things out for themselves. When parents are able to stay connected while supporting their children's separation from them, they help their children discover and develop

TABLE 7.1. Developmental Milestones in Older Teens and Young Adults (Ages 16–25)

Age	Physical	Thinking and learning	Social and emotional
16- to 18-year-olds	• Girls by 16 complete growth spurt • Boys by 16 reach peak of growth spurt; voice deepens • Boys: muscle added and body fat declines; motor performance improves • Boys complete growth spurt by 18 • May have sexual intercourse	• Decision making improves • Understands numbers can be represented in different ways: variables, fractions, decimals • Can use graphs, maps, and other mathematical representations to solve problems • Thinking becomes more abstract and reflective • May learn to drive and obtain driver's license • At 18 can register to vote (laws and rules change based on adult status in most countries)	• Explores identity • Becomes less self-conscious • Explores vocational goals and different education pathways • Moral reasoning becomes more advanced and moral standards develop • Cliques and crowds decline in importance • Mixed gender groups become common • May seek intimacy and romances that last longer • May start work and budgeting money
19- to 25-year-olds	• Development continues in the decision-making and emotion-regulation regions of the brain • Physical maturation complete; attains full height and weight	• Identifies career goals and pursues them • May learn a trade or pursue higher education • Understands abstract concepts and is aware of consequences and limitations	• Moves into adult relationship with parents • Peer groups are less important • Has better intimacy skills • Enters into sexual and emotional relationships • May have some feelings of invincibility

their purpose. Knowing and believing that their lives are valuable and serve a purpose enables them to move forward confidently in finding meaningful work that will support them while developing the relationships that will provide them with opportunities to care for and be cared for by others. (See Table 7.2 for balanced parenting with older teens and young adults.)

Going to college provides a relatively safe path for many adolescents, serving as an intermediary step between living in their parents' houses and living in their own places. Many colleges insist that students stay in a dorm or other campus housing for at least the first year, which decreases the responsibilities students have for finding a place to live, setting up utility payments, lining up transportation, and dealing with the hassles of renting an apartment or house. But many kids don't have that option, or it isn't the best one for them.

In Zack's case, he didn't know what he wanted to study and had convinced his parents that he wasn't ready for college—no easy task with two parents with doctoral degrees. But Jennifer had taught too many college students who didn't know why they were there to push him, so they agreed he would go to work instead. When she

TABLE 7.2. Balanced Parenting With Older Teens and Young Adults (Ages 16–25)

Stage and age	Developmental challenges	Balanced parenting	Resilient child outcomes
Older teens and young adults (16+)	• Identity versus conflicted	• Letting go versus staying involved	• Purpose (I have a plan; I care for myself and others)

was honest with herself, she realized that her biggest fear was not that he wouldn't figure out what he wanted to do—she had confidence that he would—but what her friends would think. Many of her friends' kids seemed to have big ambitions and were going off to prestigious universities. Clearly, it benefits our kids to put their needs ahead of worrying about how our friends might (or might not) judge us as parents.

Many teens benefit from taking some time off after high school to work, volunteer in their communities, or get jobs that give them a chance to discover where their interests lie. Parents can be supportive by keeping in touch through regular conversations if their children leave home to work or travel, trying not to ask too many questions or pressure them needlessly about their plans. When you keep your conversations positive or at least neutral (no matter how much you wish they would do what you want them to do), teens are more likely to share with you what they're learning about themselves and the directions they are thinking of going. Routine check-in conversations—such as FaceTiming every Sunday afternoon, no matter where they are or what they're doing—creates opportunities to listen with your ears and your intuition, taking note of how they're doing as well as what they're doing. When parents are nonjudgmental about relatively minor things, their almost-grown children are more likely to listen when bigger issues arise.

Parents can also help prepare their children to be ready to leave home by delegating more responsibilities to them while they are still at home. As we discussed earlier, helping them learn how to "adult" can range from teaching them to cook and store food properly, grocery shop, and manage their money to turning over responsibility for making and keeping doctor and dentist appointments on their own to taking care of their car, if they have one. When they make mistakes—as they undoubtedly will—try to see them as learning experiences and not as proof that they aren't ready for more independence or responsibility. There are some helpful books and websites in the Resources section that provide more information on helping prepare teens for adult life.

Not all young adults are ready or able to leave home by their early to mid-20s. The world has changed in the past few decades. The cost of renting apartments or houses in many major cities around the world has made renting or buying a home out of reach for many young adults. The COVID-19 pandemic also made being independent difficult for many who would normally be living on their own or with roommates. Sometimes adult children are simply afraid to leave home and need more encouragement. Some adult children with disabilities may be unable to provide for their own care or may benefit from being at home for other reasons. In these cases, giving them appropriately increasing levels of autonomy is beneficial for their mental health and development. Include them as much as possible in family decisions and avoid making decisions for them that they are able to make on their own. Some adult children return to our homes when they are in distress or their lives are in disarray. Sometimes they need assistance to recover from substance use disorders, abusive relationships, or other traumas. They may even have their own children whom they need help caring for.

Whatever the circumstances, when adult children live at home for an extended time, it is important that parents not inhibit their continued growth and development as adults. This means not continuing to treat them as children but more as adult roommates. It requires setting clear expectations about household responsibilities, communicating openly without hostility when expectations aren't met, creating a plan for the future, and working toward it. Sometimes living in multigenerational households can be beneficial to all involved, but this requires setting clear limits about using shared resources, respecting others' schedules and wishes, and solving problems and conflicts as they occur.

One of the challenges in being a supportive parent to our children as they become more independent adults is how to talk with them when we have concerns about their decisions, actions, or future plans. How do we share our (hopefully) greater experience and wisdom without disrespecting their newly acquired independence and autonomy? It turns out that there are tools for how to have conversations when the "stakes are high, opinions vary, and emotions start to run strong" (Patterson et al., 2012, p. 17). The authors of the best-selling book *Crucial Conversations* (Patterson et al., 2012) provided guidelines for how to turn these difficult situations into opportunities to understand each other better, make our relationships stronger, and solve difficult problems together. Unfortunately, most of us never learned how to have these *crucial conversations* growing up and rarely see them in action. The steps are simple, but they do require a bit of practice. We highly recommend going to the book or website for more information, but we have summarized the steps to master crucial conversations in Practical Tip 7.1: Crucial Conversations.

Practical Tip 7.1: Crucial Conversations

Conversations are "crucial" when the topic is important, opinions differ, and emotions are strong. The following steps will help you and your almost-grown child learn how to have these conversations skillfully, solving problems that would otherwise lead to arguments and can lead to stronger relationship with your child.

Step 1: Start With Heart

Ask yourself what your goals are for having the conversation. Focus on what you want—for yourself, others, and the relationship. Look for mutual purpose—how do your goals and your older teen or young adult's overlap? Search your motives, and don't assume their motives. For example,

(continues)

Practical Tip 7.1: Crucial Conversations (*Continued*)

your 20-year-old son wants to spend the summer in an apartment in his college town with his roommate. He doesn't plan to take summer classes and doesn't yet have a job there to pay for his rent and food. Think about what you want to result from the conversation. You'd like him to continue taking classes. But if not, you want him to understand he'll need to pay his expenses.

Step 2: Learn to Look

Recognize when a conversation has become crucial—that one or both of you is experiencing emotions. Signs can be physical (e.g., flushed face or neck, quickened breath), emotional (e.g., anger, fear, hurt), or behavioral (e.g., crossing arms, backing away, speaking louder). When conversations become emotional or stressful, many people use these strategies, which are the exact opposite of what works. In our example, when you tell your son that you want him to either work or go to school, he starts to look upset and says that you don't trust him to make good decisions and don't understand that he needs a break from school and stress.

Step 3: Make It Safe

Safety comes from feeling that partners have mutual purpose and respect. When you notice someone (yourself or your conversational partner) moving to either "silence or violence" (figuratively speaking), you can step out of the conversation and build safety before stepping back in. How? Decide which condition of safety is at risk: Do others believe you care about their goals in this conversation? Do others believe you respect them? Apologize if you responded in any way that left the other person feeling unsafe. If the conversation breaks down, you may need to create a new mutual purpose. In the example, you recognize that your son has become emotional, feeling like you don't respect him, so you take a deep breath and say, "I'm sorry—I didn't mean to communicate that I don't trust you. I do. You're exhausted from two tough semesters and need a break. And we both want you to be able to graduate without too much debt in student loans. How can we find a way to make that happen?"

Practical Tip 7.1: Crucial Conversations (*Continued*)

Step 4: Create a Mutual Purpose

When it seems that mutual purpose has broken down, create a new one using CRIB: Commit to finding mutual purpose (e.g., "We both want you to have a good summer that helps you get toward graduation with as little debt as possible"), recognize the purpose behind the conversation (e.g., "Tell me again why you want to stay at college this summer rather than coming home to save money?"), invent a mutual purpose (e.g., "We both want to make sure that you don't get too deeply in debt"), and brainstorm new solutions being as creative as possible (e.g., "How about we agree that you have a month to find a summer job that will let you take a break from school but pay your expenses?")

  With a little practice, you may find that the ability to have crucial conversations improves not only your relationships with your grown and nearly grown children but also with colleagues, friends, and other family members. (See the Resources section for more information.)

Balanced parenting with older teens and young adults also involves learning when to give them feedback. The world is their laboratory now—they are learning by doing (or not doing) and interacting with others outside the family. When you observe them making mistakes in their thinking, making poor choices, or acting self-destructively, allow yourself one planned and thoughtful conversation on the topic. They will not benefit from hearing it twice or again and again. As parents, you have an obligation to alert them to potential hazards and consequences they may not have seen yet, but you want them to listen and not shut out your voice. When we preach too often on the same topic, we are more likely to arouse their need to prove us wrong than to take our advice.

  However, noticing what they're doing well and commenting on it never goes amiss. We often take for granted that they are doing well, but it's nothing short of miraculous that in 2 decades, our helpless infants grow up to be capable people. Like us, they will have to learn many things the hard way and will continue to make mistakes. How well they learn and recover from those mistakes is partly up to us as parents. When we show them that we are on their side by staying calm as they fluctuate between flourishing and floundering, they can confidently go into the world and give it their best. And we can be calm because we've given them a good foundation— we provided them the relationships and resources they needed to become resilient.

PARENTING WHEN YOU HAVE ACEs: DON'T ASSUME CHILDREN WILL MAKE THE SAME MISTAKES

When parents have experienced maltreatment in their childhoods, they are more likely than parents without adverse childhood experiences (ACEs) to have made some mistakes in their adolescence— mistakes they are determined to prevent their children from making. This can lead to unbalanced parenting—being overly restrictive at one extreme or too passive at the other extreme, assuming kids will inevitably get into trouble. When parents are too restrictive or overreact to their youth's mistakes, teens are less likely to rely on their parents for advice and support for fear of getting in trouble and being punished. They begin to lie to their parents about where they are, who they are with, and what they are doing. Obviously, parents can't help them navigate the issues they are trying to handle when kids shut them out or are afraid of their reactions. You don't have to approve if you discover their risky or wrong behavior—and you should let them know when you don't approve—but you want to keep your responses from being insulting (e.g., "How could you be so stupid?"), dismissive (e.g., "I give up—do whatever you want"), or argumentative (e.g., "Why would you do such a thing?"). Again, we recommend parents spend some time learning and practicing how to talk and listen when emotions are strong, the topic is important, and opinions differ (see Practical Tip 7.1: Crucial Conversations). Remember that kids make mistakes. The most important thing is that they learn from those mistakes, which is more likely to happen when they aren't afraid to turn to you for help but instead see you as on their side and ready to help them, even when they've messed up.

At the other extreme, parents may sometimes feel like there is nothing they can do to prevent their adolescent from getting into trouble, that it's just inevitable or a part of growing up. In fact, teens will do some foolish things (e.g., "I thought I could make it home without stopping for gas," "Everyone smokes weed now that it's legal here"). As their parents, we want to prepare them beforehand to make smart decisions when they are faced with situations where it would be easy to go down the wrong path. Dinner time is a good time to informally bring up topics that would be more sensitive if they were to come up in the moment or after a mistake has been made. For example, as you're preparing or cleaning up after dinner with your 16-year-old, you can start a conversation by asking questions such as "What would you say if someone offered you a joint when you and your friends are hanging out at the park? Are you curious about how it would make you feel? Do you know why it's not a good idea for you right now—aside from it being illegal?" Our kids are much more likely to make the decisions that will keep them safe if they're prepared for situations than if they occur without having thought about them and rehearsed their responses. Again, our job as parents is not to prevent them from making any mistakes or errors in judgment—that's partly how they learn. Our job is to prepare them to make as few serious or enduring mistakes as possible and keep them from shutting us out as they learn.

One way to help you see your teenager as who they, and not you, is to write them a letter. Give them a handwritten letter before a birthday, a major transition such as graduation, or when you want to acknowledge how proud you are of them. Writing allows you to think about and express thoughts and feelings that may be difficult to say. Keep the letter positive. Focus on how you feel about them at this stage of their life. Add something about your hopes and dreams for them. It does not have to be long, but it should be specific. Remember, this is something that you can continue to do in the future when they get married or start their first job. It is easy just to text these days, but most people value having something loving and positive written in their parents' handwriting and will treasure it for years to come.

A final word about parenting older teens and young adults when we have a history of making mistakes as a result of our difficult childhoods and dysfunctional families. Sometimes we are still working through our traumas when we bring children into the world and still making some mistakes (and hopefully learning from them), and our children may have witnessed this process. Maybe we struggled to control our alcohol or drug use earlier in their childhoods. Or we brought into our family a stepparent who was harsh or abusive.

Guilt can be a powerful motivator to change, but it can also prevent us from taking a firm approach to setting limits on behavior with our teenagers. We may feel that unless we have always led blameless and perfect lives, we don't have the moral authority to tell them what to do. Or they may accuse us of being hypocritical when we tell them to do or not do something they know we did. What's a parent to do? First, remember that you can't expect them not to do something you are currently doing unless it is legal for you and not for them. But saying, "It's legal for me and not for you," will not sound like a valid reason to a 17-year-old who is eager to adopt such adult privileges as access to alcohol, so be prepared with other reasons alcohol and other drugs are detrimental to teenage brain development (for more information, see Resources). Second, be prepared to be honest about the cost of the mistakes you made. For example, you might have a conversation that begins with stating how you wish your 17-year-old self knew then what you know now. Ask them to imagine what they want to be like when they show up at their 10-year high school reunion. Helping them imagine what their future self will thank their current self for doing (or not doing) is a good way for them to get a longer term perspective on the costs and benefits of the decisions and actions they are making today.

PARENTING STRATEGIES FOR BUILDING RESILIENCE

As teens become more independent, it is important to support them in learning life skills on their own. We can do this by having conversations and listening and being available to share advice when needed or just lend an ear. When you have a good relationship with your teen, it is much easier to be a positive influence and support them in learning to be an adult. It also makes it easier to talk through mistakes when they make them. The following are some specific strategies for building resilience during this stage.

Let Them Drive

Amanda vividly remembers the first day she drove herself to high school. Unlike the mornings of the past, she was the driver, cruising along the country roads with her younger brother in the passenger seat. It was less than 10 miles to school, and she was excited to be the driver and not wait for her dad or the bus to take her to school. As she got closer to her destination, she looked in her rearview mirror. To her surprise, her father was in his pick-up truck, smiling back at her. She thought, "Surely, he is going to turn the other way, toward his office." But as she feared when she turned toward the school, so did he. In fact, he followed her all the way to the school parking lot!

Driving is one of the most dangerous activities people engage in daily. And teenage drivers are more likely to be in crashes and die than other age groups. In fact, teen drivers are almost three times as likely to have a fatal car crash as older drivers. One of the main reasons is that they are less experienced drivers. They are also more likely to engage in more risky driving when they are with their friends. So, it's a good idea to give your teens lots of opportunities to practice driving while you are with them. That way, they get to practice, and you can give them feedback. It goes without saying that it is important for parents to remain calm when their kids are learning to drive (easier said than done!), but wouldn't you rather that your children learn to drive while you are there to provide guidance rather than learn later from someone else?

Many states in the United States have regulations that provide for a permit year when teens can only drive with their parents or another fully licensed adult family member. We recommend taking full advantage of the permit year. Let your children do most of the driving during this period to get as much experience as possible. Also, be grateful for the driver's ed teachers who provide driving lessons! When you live in the city, it can be difficult to find a place to allow your teens to practice driving, but empty parking lots and getting outside of the city are great ideas for those first-time driving experiences ("Now which one is the brake, and which one is the gas?" Didn't all those driving video games at least help them out a bit?)

Monitoring: Talking and Listening

As we talked about in Chapter 6, it is important for parents to know where their teens are, who they are with, and how they are spending their time and money. When teens first start driving, make rules together and decide on a curfew and consequences for breaking the rules. When they get home from being out, have them check in with you and casually look for signs of substance use. As we discussed in Chapter 6, if you smell alcohol on their breath or marijuana on their clothes, wait until the morning to talk about it. Experimentation is normal in our society, but regular usage is problematic, especially when teens are still in high school. Research has shown that teens whose parents have rules regarding drinking and drug use are less likely to abuse alcohol and illegal substances. It may be tempting to ignore substance use as teens get older or to allow them to drink at home, but this will likely lead to more usage.

When parents use and abuse substances, teens are more likely to do so as well. Having rules about not doing anything illegal or harmful is a good idea. Be honest and direct—for example, "We do not do illegal things in our home, and it is not yet legal for you to drink alcohol," or "It may be legal for adults to use marijuana, but we don't believe it helps us or think it's good for you because your brain is still developing." Adolescence is a good time for parents to check their alcohol consumption in front of their kids, show responsible behavior, and consider cutting back if you think it may be a good idea for you to do so.

It is also critical to have rules and conversations about substance use and driving—that it is never allowed, and children should always be able to call you for a ride or use a rideshare program such as Uber or Lyft when they are old enough to do so. Risks regarding substance use and other behaviors should be discussed, too. Teens are more likely to engage in unprotected sex and mix substances when they are drinking alcohol. Having honest conversations about risks, healthy behavior (using protection, not mixing substances, protecting your drink at a party from someone putting something in it) makes a difference. As with other conversations, don't make it one big talk. Rather, have multiple conversations when topics come up and make it okay for teens to talk with you and ask questions. And listen to what they have to say.

Most teens engage in risky behaviors because it satisfies some need they have, usually to fit in with their peers or to feel more independent and grown up. And most adolescents underestimate the risks and overestimate the benefits of behaviors such as drinking and driving. Giving them opportunities to talk about these issues and listening to them without overreacting is important but is not always easy. Be sure to find out why they are experimenting with substances because there may be an underlying mental health issue, such as depression or anxiety, and they are self-medicating (see Chapter 6 for more on this). These conversations are likely to provoke some strong feelings. But learning to talk and listen to your teens and young adults when the stakes are high, opinions differ, and emotions are strong is a valuable skill that will benefit both you and your child in the future.

As adolescents mature and leave home, how parents monitor their behavior should change. It is tempting to track your children using modern apps to see if they are attending class, at a fraternity party, or at the concert they told you they were going to, but monitoring when you have no control will just make you worry. When kids leave home, set a regular time to talk by phone or FaceTime. Check in regularly and ask how things are going. If possible, plan some weekend trips to see them, meet their friends, and show them that you're interested and intend to stay connected and supportive of them.

Help Them Prepare for Adulthood

There are many things that parents can do to help their teens and young adults prepare for living on their own. One way is to increase their responsibilities at home—have them do their laundry, make their breakfast or lunch, and help cook dinner. Most teens enjoy planning and preparing meals for the family. Helping them make a grocery list and shop for food can be a great way for a teen to gain independence, help the family, and learn about living on a budget. The idea of teens not being ready to live on their own when they leave home and having difficulty "adulting" likely comes from parents doing too much for their kids. Amanda knows of one 17-year-old who was at the doctor's office on his own for a routine visit. The mom had checked, and it was fine for him to go alone because he had been there before. When filling out the usual visit paperwork, the teen called his mom to ask, "What is a dob?" His mother was confused at first, then said, "You mean D-O-B, date of birth?" None of us know what we don't know, so giving teens a chance to begin learning what they don't know while we're still around them is a good way to help them become ready for that big step. There are some good books for both parents and teens on how to ensure that your kids are prepared to take care of themselves when they leave home and how to take on a reasonable share of household chores before they do (see Resources at the end of the chapter)!

Identity development does not suddenly end when one turns 18 but is ongoing into young adulthood. In fact, we continue to explore our identities throughout our lives as our roles change—when we become a parent, get a new job or start a different career, get married, become a grandparent, or lose a spouse through divorce or death. Nevertheless, adolescence and young adulthood is the first time we develop a coherent identity, making it an important time for youth to explore who they are. What do they want to do in their lives? What do they want to be like in the future? How are their values and goals different from those of their parents? Parents can help by having conversations and being open to their teens' ideas, goals, and beliefs, especially if they differ from their own (see Zooming In 7.2: Forming an Identity).

Zooming In 7.2: Forming an Identity

The formation of a stable and coherent identity—knowing one's career path, values, and life goals—is one of the primary tasks of adolescence. Adolescents may go down several paths to accomplish this task. One path, *identity achievement*, occurs when the teen or young adult has actively explored different careers, goals, and values and makes a commitment to an identity. A second path, *identity moratorium*, occurs when they are still exploring ideas and options but have a low commitment to any particular identity. This is common in teenagers but can be distressing if this indecision continues well into adulthood. A third path, *identity foreclosure*, occurs when teens or young adults commit to a set of goals or values or career path without exploring any other options, usually because of pressure from their parents or others. They may "wake up" in midlife and realize they've never been happy with their career or other life choices. The fourth path, *identity diffusion*, occurs when teens or young adults have a low commitment to an identity and low motivation to explore different options. They may be overwhelmed by choices (too many or too few) or suffer from depression or other conditions that prevent them from exploring and deciding on a career, values, or goals.

Parents can help their youth move into identity achievement by not putting too much pressure on them to decide (foreclosure), helping them explore their options (moratorium), and helping them find ways to explore when they appear to lack ideas or the confidence to check out their options (diffusion). When parents are able to support their children's exploration and decisions by letting go while staying involved, their adolescents and young adults are more likely to discover their purpose and create an independent life caring for others as well as themselves (Marcia, 1966).

As we discuss later in this chapter, it is important for us to keep supporting our children and being their advocates. We can do this by being available, listening, keeping communication open, and spending time together. When adolescents officially become adults, legally their status changes, and their parents are no longer their legal guardians. It is important to talk about what this means—that teens are responsible for their behavior legally, and there can be different consequences. As teens become more responsible—having a job, managing their own money, and being in a committed relationship—important conversations can help them handle challenges and opportunities that may arise. Providing a supportive, listening environment is key, particularly when young adults are struggling. Basic financial literacy and budgeting are difficult for adolescents to learn until they have their own money and financial discretion, but it is never too early to talk about the importance of saving, giving, and planning for the future (see Practical Tip 7.2: Talking About Money).

Practical Tip 7.2: Talking About Money

Amanda's husband, Mike, is an economist. She asked him what the most important advice was to give parents to help them teach their kids about money. He said, "Teach them to save. Don't save to buy something later; just save to save." Teach them to always save at least 10% of everything they earn. Parents can help their kids set up a savings account and might consider paying them interest on what they save. This gives them just a small amount as an incentive to save. Kids should also be encouraged to set aside money for charity or a cause that is important to them. Around the holidays, when families are giving gifts to one another, it is good to remember to also give to others. Basic budgeting is important, too. Let kids know how much the cell phone, car insurance, and other expenses cost so they can appreciate money. It is important to have them cover some expenses, too, such as gas and entertainment. Another strategy you may find helpful is to split costs with your teens on things that are not necessities (e.g., a new phone or new shoes for prom). This gives them a stake in things and helps them realize the value of money. It is good for teens to have a job, but remember that schoolwork comes first. It is a balancing act to be sure kids are getting what they need from school and activities while also working a part-time job during the school year or a full-time job in the summer.

PARENTING OLDER TEENS AND YOUNG ADULTS
WHO HAVE A HISTORY OF ACEs

One of the most difficult aspects of parenting is realizing that because of our ACEs or other life experiences, and despite our best intentions and efforts to protect our children, they may have experienced adversity or trauma. Dealing with our guilt or shame that we were not able to keep ACEs out of our children's lives is the first step in helping them recover. When we're dealing with our emotions and needs, we are not able to focus on our children's needs. If these feelings are overwhelming, talk with a professional about them. Mental health professionals are increasingly being trained to use trauma-informed practices—recognizing issues that have their roots in childhood trauma and how to take steps to recover and heal from it. The next thing to do is to become trauma-informed yourself. Being trauma-informed involves realizing the widespread effects of trauma and understanding paths to recovery, recognizing the signs and symptoms of trauma in our children and other family members and responding by applying what we have learned about the availability of resources to support our children and help them recover. Posttraumatic growth can be the goal of parents and children who've experienced trauma in their families, using their experiences as opportunities to make meaning from the past and build stronger supports for the future.

Older adolescents and young adults are more likely to experience mental health issues today than at any time in history. Research published before the COVID-19 pandemic showed that mood disorders (such as depression and anxiety) and suicide-related outcomes increased significantly between 2013 and 2019, with nearly one out of five (19%) high school students having seriously considered suicide in 2019 (Bitsko et al., 2022). Social media was suggested as one likely cause of this increase, as well as declining rates of sleep duration in this age group. Social media can be damaging to teens' mental health because they may make unrealistic comparisons with others and are exposed to cyberbullying, which has been linked to depression and self-harm, particularly in girls.

In a 2021 survey of high school students, those who reported having four or more ACEs during the COVID-19 pandemic were a staggering 25 times more likely to report suicidal behaviors (Anderson et al., 2022). These alarming statistics suggest that we are just beginning to understand the effects of the pandemic on teens and young adults. Certainly, parents of older adolescents and young adults have observed and experienced the effects of their children's isolation from their peers and the disruption of normal rites of passage (e.g., high school proms, graduation, going away to school, leaving home to live with roommates). It is safe to say that the COVID-19 pandemic will be a defining experience for our children who came of age during this time, one that may have long-term effects on their mental health and well-being.

As we discussed in Chapter 6, parents can help by being aware of changes in their teen or young adult's behavior, sleep or eating habits, interest in usual activities or friends, or use of alcohol or other substances. These changes often signal the onset of depression, anxiety, or other mental health problems, and the earlier they receive support and assistance from a mental health professional, the less likely it is that these problems will worsen or persist (for more specific information on symptoms and getting help, see Chapter 6). It is important to note, too, that these experiences can build resilience. Going through difficult times helps us learn to cope and be stronger when future adversity occurs.

We hope you have developed an appreciation for the power of protective and compensatory experiences (PACEs) to help you parent your child with ACEs and build resilience as you have read previous chapters and started to add more PACEs to your own and your family's routines. We want to emphasize in this chapter the unique importance of one PACE for older teens and young adults: physical activity. Physical activity has been described as a universal depression prevention strategy in young people. Encouraging and supporting our adolescents to get regular physical activity is one of the most important things we can do to support their health. Being physically active improves brain health; improves bone, cardiovascular, and metabolic functioning; improves cognition; and decreases the risk of depression. Physical activity can include a wide range of exercises, including aerobic (running, brisk walking, cycling, doing martial arts), muscle-strengthening (weightlifting, resistance training), balance (wobble boards, yoga), and flexibility (stretching, yoga) activities. Encourage your teen to find at least one activity they enjoy alone or with others. Think creatively if they don't enjoy traditional exercises. Dance, rock climbing, and other active sports such as swimming, basketball, and tennis are also good options that can be enjoyed throughout adulthood. Most important, walk the talk! Find activities that get you moving and you enjoy. There is no better way to manage stress, stay healthy, improve cognitive skills, and prevent depression.

KEY TAKEAWAYS

As in other chapters, we provide a summary of the most important tips we have for building resilience in older adolescents and young adults:

- Don't assume your children will make the same mistakes you made as an adolescent. It is important not to be overly protective or give up on your teen because you think you cannot make a difference. Our children are their own persons on their own journeys. We cannot control them, but we can be an important influence in their lives.

- Stay connected. Are you checking in and staying involved in your teen's life without being too intrusive? Keep lines of communication open and accept the person your child is becoming. Respect their need for privacy and autonomy.
- Provide opportunities that help your adolescent become more of an adult. Allow them to practice being an adult while they are still at home by encouraging them to go to appointments on their own, get a part-time job, have a bank account, make dinner, grocery shop, do their own laundry, and do other household tasks.
- Keep listening. It is important to have rules and continue to monitor behavior, particularly when teens start driving. However, as adolescents mature, have conversations regularly and stay involved rather than creating and attempting to enforce rules. Offer choices, not demands, and acknowledge responsibilities, and praise teens when they are doing well.
- Walk your talk. Be the example of the adult you want your children to become, whether it is how you treat others, manage your time and money, use moderation in eating and drinking, be physically active, set goals for yourself, and flexibly adjust them as conditions change. Your kids have always paid more attention to what you do than what you say, and now they are watching more carefully than ever. You are the best role model they will ever have.
- Recognize that they may make the same mistakes you did—and probably some you didn't think of—so try to avoid being either obsessively protective or hopelessly detached. Aim for being trusting but watchful. Assume they are doing their best, but realize they aren't fully prepared for the challenges life will throw them. They will make mistakes. Mistakes were often our greatest teachers, and mistakes likely have lessons in store for our offspring. But by being on their side and preparing

them as much as possible, you can help them avoid the truly costly mistakes and learn from the rest.

ACTIVITIES: YOU ARE HERE

Now, take a minute to think about where you are with balancing the competing demands of letting go and staying involved. Are you aware of your teen's activities, and are they involved in making decisions about rules and consequences? For young adults, do you know how your child is doing, and are you having regular check-ins and conversations? Are you supporting them as they make decisions about their life direction? The following are some other general questions to ponder:

- What am I doing well as a parent? What do I like most about my adolescent or young adult? What do I enjoy most about parenting my child at this age? What is something we still enjoy doing together?
- What PACEs do I currently have? Are there PACEs that I need to develop? If so, which ones? What is my plan for encouraging PACEs for my adolescent or young adult? Getting enough physical activity is essential at this age, but are there other PACEs I can encourage and support?
- Do I need to find professional help for my child or myself? Are there signs that my child is struggling and may have anxiety, depression, or a substance use problem? It is never too late to seek help; it can be life saving for a teen.

Expressive Writing

For more than 30 years, thousands of people with traumatic experiences have become happier and healthier using a simple technique called expressive writing (Pennebaker, 2018). We have seen that having ACEs can increase the chances of having serious physical and mental health problems. Dr. Jamie Pennebaker and his colleagues at the University of Texas discovered that one of the reasons for these health problems is not the trauma itself but the act of keeping it secret. When we run from the problem or actively prevent ourselves from thinking about or sharing it, we put another layer of stress on ourselves. Expressive writing helps because it gives us an opportunity to create a story about ourselves where we integrate the trauma and stress into a bigger story. In the larger story, not only do we encounter adversity but we also survive it, begin to recover, and continue to recover. Writers often discover that in their stories are elements of resilience and heroism, lessons learned, opportunities found, and feelings of gratitude and awe that accompany the memories of fear, shame, and loss.

Many people find the exercise emotionally upsetting and may be sad or depressed for a few days. You may be tempted to stop after a day or two, but we encourage you to press on. The benefits come from completing the process. But the overwhelming majority of people find it valuable and meaningful in their lives. And the research is clear that it leads to improved physical and mental health outcomes. We invite you to follow the instructions to see what expressive writing might hold for you.

Expressive Writing Instructions[1]

For the next 3 to 5 days, find a time and place where you can write without interruption for 20 minutes. Think a little about where you feel comfortable writing. Some people like to be alone, and others

---

[1]This section was adapted from Pennebaker (2018).

prefer being surrounded by others sitting in a booth of a bustling coffee shop or at a quiet table in the public library. Choose your place, get comfortable with a pen and plenty of paper, and set a timer for 20 minutes. Then begin writing about your deepest thoughts and feelings about an extremely emotional issue that has affected you and your life. The topic might be your relationships with others, including parents, lovers, friends, or relatives. It might be about your past, present, or future or who you have been, are now, or would like to be. As you write, just let the words come. Allow yourself to go wherever your thoughts take you. As you write, do not worry about spelling, sentence structure, or grammar. No one else ever needs to read what you write. The only rule is that once you begin writing, continue writing until 20 minutes is up.

The next day, you may continue to write about the same topic or choose another one. If after 5 days you still have things to write about, you may want to start keeping a journal to write in as thoughts and insights come up. Many people find it beneficial to keep a record of how the process unfolds over time. Be prepared to observe how becoming aware of your deepest thoughts and feelings affects your outlook afterward, your relationships, and the choices you make in the future. You may also find it helpful to talk with a psychologist or other trained professional as you accept and integrate experiences or parts of yourself that before were kept closed.

RESOURCES

Parenting Older Teens and Young Adults

Faber, A., & Mazlish, E. (2006). *How to talk so teens will listen and listen so teens will talk*. William Morrow.

Lythcott-Haims, J. (2015). *How to raise an adult: Break free of the over-parenting trap and prepare your kid for success*. Holt.

Ray, B. (2019, October 21). How to help young people transition into adulthood. *Greater Good Magazine.* https://greatergood.berkeley.edu/article/item/how_to_help_young_people_transition_into_adulthood

Steinberg, L. (2023). *You and your adult child: How to grow together in challenging times.* Simon & Schuster.

Automobile Safety

See https://www.apa.org/monitor/2022/09/hazard-perception-teen-drivers for more information on how psychology-informed interventions help keep teen drivers safe.

Preventing and Treating Alcohol and Drug Use in Adolescents and Young Adults

Centers for Disease Control and Prevention. (2022). *Why drinking less matters.* https://www.cdc.gov/drinklessbeyourbest/drinking_less_matters.html?s_cid=NCCDPHP_google_search_drinkless_consequences_uc

Hopson, J. (2016, May 1). How alcohol ravages the teen brain. *Scientific American.* https://www.scientificamerican.com/article/how-alcohol-ravages-the-teen-brain/

Expressive Writing

Pennebecker, J., & Smyth, J. (2016). *Opening up by writing it down: How expressive writing improves health and eases emotional pain.* Guilford Press.

Books for Your Adolescent or Young Adult

Morin, A. (2021). *Adulting made easy: Things someone should have told you about getting your grown-up act together.* Sixth & Spring Books.

Newman, C. (2020). *How to be a person: 65 hugely useful super-important skills to learn before you're grown up.* Storey.

CHAPTER 8

BEING A RESILIENT PARENT: IT'S ALL ABOUT BALANCE!

It was the fall of 2020, and the COVID-19 pandemic had been going on for 6 months. Amanda's 15- and 17-year-old children were in high school online, and it felt anything but natural to keep them home all the time. There was no going out with friends and no after-school activities. There were no vaccines, and there was a lot of worry. The family was around Amanda's husband Mike's aging parents, and Amanda was having some health problems, so they were strict about following the guidelines, staying outside when talking with neighbors or friends, wearing masks, and using hand sanitizer. Everyone in Amanda's household was on a different schedule. The kids were staying up late, and Amanda and Mike were teaching a mix of in-person and online classes at the university. In another state, Amanda's father's health was declining rapidly, and it became obvious that her parents would soon need to move into assisted living. Amanda's son was applying to colleges, but they didn't know what it would look like when it was time for him to go. The "sandwich generation" (those caring for both the older and younger generations at the same time) was real. When asked how she was, Amanda would respond that she was hanging on by her fingernails. She had support and resources and knew the pandemic was causing hardships much greater for many families. But, still, it was challenging to get up every day and keep going.

Across the globe, we have all learned a great deal about surviving the difficult times brought about by the COVID-19 pandemic. Personally, we have witnessed how adversity can strike when we least expect it and that the way to be resilient is to be prepared with habits, attitudes, and knowledge. We drew on the support and assistance of friends and family and gained a new appreciation for the resources available in our communities. And as our children have grown and started their own lives, we have learned that parenting changes but never ends. In this chapter, we summarize and highlight the most important lessons we have learned.

BALANCED PARENTING

Being a parent is lifelong. When our children are little, we look forward to the days when they can brush their own teeth, make themselves a snack, and control the impulse to hit their sibling when they take their favorite toy. Parenting is physically demanding and time-consuming, and we can't even imagine these same children someday setting the alarm and getting themselves up, dressed, and off to school. When our children reach that much-anticipated stage, we discover they still need us, but now they need us to help them figure out more demanding challenges, such as how to manage their time when homework and an after-school job conflict, what to do when their friends begin to experiment with drugs, what they should do with their lives after high school, or . . . well, the list is nearly endless. Then we realize that parenting is never really over. We may get to a point where we think they'll be fine if something happened to us, that they have the foundation for making good decisions and moving forward with their lives. But we also know how helpful it can be to have an older, hopefully, wiser, and more experienced adult who is always on their side and ready to be supportive no matter what they encounter. Being a balanced parent across a lifetime means continuing to be available for emotional support, information, and advice, regardless of their age.

Balanced parenting involves staying calm when strong emotions would otherwise jeopardize common sense or derail good decisions. When children are young, it is relatively simple. If we can remember that someone must be the grown-up in the room, and that person is us, we can usually remind ourselves to take a deep breath before responding in anger and think before taking action to manage situations. Fortunately, as our children develop and gain experience, so do we. By the time our children become adolescents or young adults with more complex problems and challenging decisions to make, we have also gained experience and wisdom. If we have been consciously developing our communication skills, learning about ourselves, gaining control over negative thoughts and feelings, and forming supportive relationships with others, we have become more resilient. We are prepared to cope with adversity and help our children cope when they encounter difficulties. Here, we emphasize three strategies that build resilience in parents, regardless of the age of their child.

Stay Calm

At the risk of repeating ourselves, we emphasize the importance of parents learning and using what psychologists refer to as *emotion regulation* skills. Think about the examples we provided in Chapter 2 when we talked about how adversity and stress can change the way our brains develop, causing us to react to stressful situations with fight, flight, or freeze responses and preventing us from thinking rationally, reacting calmly, or connecting with others who can provide help and support. The opposite response to fight–flight–freeze is to be composed and alert. The initial fight–flight–freeze response is like the smoke alarm that goes off when the oil in the pan on the stove begins to smoke. It alerts you that there is a problem. Alarms can save our kitchens and even our lives. But if the alarm continues to go off even after the danger is gone, it is no longer useful. In fact, if an alarm constantly beeps or shrieks every time water is boiled and steam rises, you may be tempted to throw it away and live without an alarm. Like a malfunctioning smoke alarm, childhood trauma may cause our bodies to either overreact or fail to react when threats are perceived.

Balanced parenting avoids being either too reactive or indifferent to the warning signs of problems. Sometimes this requires us to rewire our internal alarm system, making an effort and taking the time to learn how to control our responses. One of the most effective ways to do this is to practice mindfulness, finding some time to be alone and present, focusing on our breathing, and letting our thoughts enter and leave our consciousness without judgment or emotion. It sounds easy, but there is a reason we call it "practicing" mindfulness. Like any other skill, when we practice remaining calm, nonreactive, and nonjudgmental—no matter what painful memories or malicious thoughts come up to consciousness—we gain mastery and control over our thoughts, our emotions, and ourselves. As we gain this ability, we become more capable of navigating the challenges and difficulties that arise in our lives and the lives of our children.

Throughout history, meditation, prayer, and spirituality have provided people with the strength to cope and remain positive and calm during adversity and times of stress. Studies have shown that being spiritual is associated with better physical and mental health. Many find a calmness in formal and informal religious practices. In addition to providing a source of calm or meaning during troubled times, being active in a faith-based or spiritual community can also provide opportunities to learn through study groups, volunteer and help others, and make friends who share values and interests and support each other during times of hardship. Bringing someone a casserole after a death in their family or sitting with a friend in the hospital are acts of kindness that mean a lot when someone is suffering. As we've seen in our discussions about volunteering, we also benefit when we act out of kindness and concern for others, perhaps as much as those we are helping.

Faith can be tricky—it is uniquely personal, and what provides meaning and support to one person may rekindle painful memories of bad experiences in someone else. But the evidence is clear that having a source of strength is enormously helpful in coping with adversity. You may not have found a philosophical or belief system that gives you strength and purpose yet, but it may be helpful. The happiest people are those who have discovered a way to be at peace with themselves and the mysteries of life, whether it conforms to an accepted religion or philosophy or something of their own making. There are a number of ways to find a group you feel a sense of belonging and attachment to. Many people find "their people" through volunteering—at animal rescue organizations, food banks, or their local schools or through hobbies or sports. Avoiding the pain of loneliness is one of the ways we can create more calmness and well-being in our lives, especially as our children get older and begin to lead lives that are more separate from ours.

Focus on the Relationship

Parents who focus on keeping the relationships with their children strong are better able to help them deal with adversity. The balancing act this requires is staying on their side while also staying in your role as their parent—staying in your lane. Jennifer remembers her kids trying to get an extra hour of play before bedtime by saying, "Please, please, please—I'll be your best friend." Her response was always the same: "Sorry—I'm your mom, not your best friend." It may be tempting at times to be a best friend and play another round or two of Uno, but our children need us to stay in the parent role.

Parents or caregivers who take on the parenting role provide something unique in their children's lives: unconditional love, guidance, and feedback. We do not withhold love from children when they make mistakes, but we are also obliged to help them avoid and recover from problems when they occur. Love should not be contingent or based on behavior or performance. Parents must actively communicate that they love their children, no matter what. This is the foundation for parent–child attachment, which we discussed in Chapter 3. Children need to know they can always go to their parents for help, advice, and support. As children get older, they need to know that parents have their backs and love them even if they do not agree with all the choices they make. This can be communicated through deliberate conversations as well as through simple actions, such as delighting in your child when they do well on a test they were worried about, you make an especially tasty dinner together, or you give them your full attention when they have something they want to talk about.

Unconditional love is not the same as unconditional approval. There are many situations when parents are compelled to correct their children's behavior. In fact, it often seems that all we do is give them direction and feedback, from "Don't hit your sister" and "Put away your toys" in toddlerhood to "Do your homework before playing video games" and "You forgot to hang up your towel after your bath again" in middle childhood to "It is past your bedtime" and "Text me when you arrive at your friend's house" in adolescence. As they get older and the consequences of their mistakes can be more serious, providing unconditional love as well as rules, guidelines, and feedback becomes even more important. It is helpful to occasionally remind yourself and your growing children that you will always love them even if you don't love what they do. When your relationship is strong and mostly filled with positive interactions, your children are more likely to listen to you and your advice when it is critical. In fact, it increases the chances that you will have a positive influence on their decisions for the rest of their lives.

Trust Yourself and Learn From Others

Another balancing act resilient parents have acquired is learning when to trust their instincts and intuition and when they need help from others. The most famous child-rearing expert of the 20th century, Dr. Benjamin Spock, became well known for reminding the new mothers of the 1950s that they knew more than they thought they did and should trust their instincts (Spock, 1957). While there is a lot of value in this advice, we know now that our instinctive responses to our children's behavior (and misbehavior) are not always best. This is especially true when our parents were not the kind of parents we would have liked them to be. When we are trying to break cycles of adversity or apply different principles (e.g., using discipline rather than punishment) in raising our children, it can be helpful to seek advice from other parents, take a parenting class, or talk with a family therapist. Otherwise, we might be tempted just to do the opposite of our parents—if they were too harsh or punitive, we may be tempted to be too lenient and permissive; if they were neglectful and uninvolved, we might err on the side of being overprotective.

While going with our instincts or "trusting our gut response" is not always advised, neither is ignoring our own intelligent and intuitive observations. As balanced parents, we recognize that we are always learning but that we are the experts on our children. We know them, their temperaments and needs, their likes and dislikes. We know how they will likely respond to our expectations and feedback, and we trust ourselves to act with love and kindness. We also recognize that we can benefit from learning better ways to talk, listen, and care for them. Parenting is indeed a lifelong job and a lifelong learning experience!

PARENTING WHEN YOU HAVE ACEs: FIVE STEPS FOR BREAKING THE CYCLE OF ACEs

Throughout the book, we have created a pathway for you and the children you are raising or helping to raise to become more resilient and better equipped to survive and grow after adversity. We assume that adversity has either already occurred in your life or theirs or that it can occur at any time in the future. We hope that you have been following along as we've discussed the steps to resilience. Like the superhero who undergoes trauma and emerges with superpowers— but still has to learn how to use them—the activities we have invited you to do throughout the book will help you strengthen those resilience muscles.

We build resilience by increasing our knowledge, creating new attitudes and habits, and acquiring new skills. You may have already realized that by creating these new resilience muscles, you are doing your part to break the cycle of adversity. The long-term effects of adverse childhood experiences (ACEs) are like invisible chains that prevent parents from breaking free of intergenerational patterns, preventing them from protecting their children from ACEs or teaching them how to overcome them. But these chains can be broken. The following steps, like protective and compensatory experiences (PACEs), are simple but require some practice.

Acknowledge Your Past

The first step is acknowledging both the good and the bad of your childhood and adolescence. Most people with ACEs have spent a good part of their life trying to outrun them. One of the ways human beings cope with pain is by denial. If the pain was intense enough, we might even have separated ourselves from the experience while it was happening, which is called *dissociation*. Without a lot of support, including professional help, those experiences may be difficult to recall and acknowledge. We do not advocate reliving experiences (except under professional guidance), but we do know that the way forward is to stop running. Thousands of people have begun the process of becoming resilient by acknowledging their past, their ACEs, and their PACEs. Recognize that ACEs likely didn't start with you, and trace your family's history of adversity and the protective factors that helped them survive using the ACEs and PACEs genograms.

This is a good time to have conversations with your family members about the past. Talk with them about what happened as compassionately and nonjudgmentally as possible. See if you can understand their perspectives; parents and other family members often have a history of trauma, too. In addition, it is helpful to reflect on the "ghosts" and "angels" in our childhoods—the conscious or unconscious memories of either harsh attitudes and hurtful actions or the words and deeds of people who let us know we were loved and cared for. These are the patterns we inherit from our parents and grandparents, keeping the intergenerational legacy of adversity— or resilience—alive and active. (See ACEs and PACEs surveys in Chapter 2 and ACEs and PACEs genograms in Chapter 3.)

Manage Your Emotions

The second step, introduced in Chapter 4, is learning how to recognize and manage our emotions so that strong feelings don't lead to reacting without thinking but allow us to respond with intention and presence of mind. We recommend that parents spend a few minutes every day or two practicing *mindfulness*, the ability to observe and notice the thoughts and emotions that are constantly going through our minds, using a variety of mindful meditations. Parents who master their emotions through mindfulness are able to express their feelings appropriately and react to their children's emotional outbursts in a calm, responsive way.

Research has shown that practicing mindfulness, even for a short while, helps us manage stress better, sleep better, and be physically healthier. Parents who practice mindfulness find it easier to be fully present and listen to others with their full attention. They stay calm but also recognize their emotions and the emotions of their children. They are compassionate toward themselves and their children, remembering that the relationship with their child is what is most important. This practice is the best way to reprogram your brain from the fight, fight, or flee response and remain calm when stressed. (See Mindful Meditations activity in Chapter 4.)

Identify Outgrown Coping Strategies

The third step in breaking the cycle of adversity is to identify the coping strategies we began using when we were young to survive the stress and pain of ACEs. These survival strategies, or childhood adaptations to ACEs (ChAACEs), once served an important role in our lives. They may have kept our misery at bay, prevented others from pitying us or treating us differently, or allowed us to channel our attention and energy into getting into better circumstances. Some ChAACEs are positive: seeking help from other adults or distancing yourself from a dysfunctional family through schoolwork, sports, or other outside activities.

Some ChAACEs may have short-term benefits, such as dissociation or acting in the parental role to keep your home life from completely falling apart, but they can be harmful when used in the long run. And some ChAACEs are frankly harmful even in the short term, though they may still have helped you survive at the time. Examples of these negative adaptations to trauma include using alcohol or other substances, avoiding being with others, or cutting or other types of self-harming.

Parents who want to break the cycle of adversity are able to recognize whether the strategies they used as children have followed them into adulthood. Are there strategies that are still beneficial to you? Perhaps you go for a run when you're stressed or call an older and wiser friend for advice when you're struggling with a problem. These are positive and healthy ways to cope. Perhaps you are still avoiding your feelings by working long hours, drinking or eating too much, or avoiding being close to others. Now is a good time to look at the strategies you are using. As they get older, your children are likely to imitate your strategies for coping when they are stressed. (See the ChAACEs activity in Chapter 5.)

Develop Positive Adult Coping Strategies

After you have identified any ChAACEs that have followed you into adulthood and decided which ones to keep, modify, or discard, you are already halfway into the fourth step: choosing the grown-up adaptations to ACEs (GrAACEs) that you want to use to manage stress and cope with adversity and model for your children. Remember that you are not to blame for the ChAACEs your childhood self used to survive. In fact, we can be grateful for ChAACEs helping us to survive. Our challenge as parents breaking the cycle of adversity is to choose wisely the coping strategies we use now and that our children are learning from us. Some of our old strategies may still be beneficial or need a little updating. But developing new strategies will likely pay off for your mental health and well-being, as well as for your effectiveness as a parent.

Children are apt to "do as we do" rather than as we say. As you think about potential ways you could be managing stress, we encourage you to spend a little time thinking about the life you want to live. Consider the kind of atmosphere you want to create in your home and the patterns, habits, and traditions your responses to stress and difficulties can support. For example, if you learn to manage your stress through mindful meditation and create a system to call a family meeting when a problem arises that affects others, you are likely to find that the whole family begins to deal with problems when they are small, before anyone is too upset and every family member wants to be involved in helping solve the problem.

Recognize That Your Children Are Different From You

The final step in breaking the cycle of adversity in the next generation is not to assume that your children will make the same mistakes you did. One of the greatest gifts we can give our children is truly seeing them as themselves. They are not us. Nor are they their other parent or our crazy Uncle Ed or whoever they sometimes remind us of (and fear they are too much like). In Chapter 7, we described how seeing them as they are can prevent us from being either overprotective ("I know what I was up to at that age") or fatalistic and underinvolved ("All the kids I knew did that"). When we make an effort to listen and see how they are both similar and different from us, we give them permission to be themselves, and we can tailor our rules and support to fit them. We help them become more resilient when we give them permission and space to become the best they can be.

STRATEGIES FOR RESILIENCE

Remember the idea of the road map, the epic parenting journey? We come back to that analogy, highlighting some of the most vital concepts that apply across different stages of childhood and parenting.

None of these ideas are new, but they capture some of the most important messages we want to convey.

Enjoy the Ride

We talked about the importance of cherishing each stage of your child's life. Children are only that age once, but you will always be their parent. There are magical moments that parents can miss if they don't take the time to notice how their children are growing and maturing. Putting away the newborn onesies is something most of us remember, as well as waiting in line with our teens for the driver's license exam. Suddenly, we realize how time slips away. When they are young, one of the best things we can do is just be with them. Look at the world through their eyes, following their gaze and realizing their wonder at seeing lights and shadows, colors, and objects all around them. As they begin to play and use their imagination, jump in, and follow along with their stories; never mind that the logic is absurd, and horses don't fly. As they get older, find ways to be interested in their interests, activities, hopes, and dreams.

One way to stay engaged and present is by unplugging regularly. Certainly, you should do so at bedtime and family meals, but also consider a day or an afternoon on the weekend and several times a year on family vacations. This is good to model for our kids, and everyone benefits when we learn how to put our phones away and focus on each other. Teens like to say, "Hang up and hang out." This is great advice! Old-fashioned family game nights can be great fun. Teaching kids how to play card games is good for their mental development (counting, matching, learning probabilities) and helps them learn how to win and lose in a safe environment. Games and play are great ways for parents and kids to feel connected and build up a store of positive memories. Creating these routines keeps us on track even when difficulties arise. Like riding a bike, we keep our balance when we keep moving, even when the road is rocky or wet.

Change Directions

Most people have experienced a road trip when the GPS interrupted the drive with the "Recalculating" screen. This happens when we make a wrong turn or when the road maps and highway information are out of date in the system. Sometimes as parents, we need to recalculate where we are headed and adjust our expectations. On the parenting road trip, we switch from being the driver to teaching our kids to drive to eventually letting them drive the car while we nap in the passenger seat or allow them to take the trip on their own. It is easy for parents to expect their children to be just like them or like their ideal image of who they wish they were. Indeed, many parents live their lives through their children. In some ways, it can be nice to relive important milestones. But parents have to be careful not to overly influence children, to try to create the childhood or adolescence they wish they could have had. A mom might wish she could have been a cheerleader, so she pushes her child to try out for the cheerleading team. Or a parent might have always wanted to go to medical school, so they push their teen into Advanced Placement science and biology classes in high school. All of this is fine if their children also want these things. Parents need to watch out for this because it is natural to think that our kids want what we wanted when we were their age. But most children have their own ideas.

In fact, our children may be different from us at birth. One way they may differ from us is in their *temperaments*, their biological predispositions toward different reactions to the world. As infants, they may be easily consoled or difficult to soothe. As young children, they may be naturally withdrawn and shy or gregarious and the life of the party. Parents have to observe their children and learn what works best according to their children's temperament. Some children respond well when given choices and variety, while others respond better to having set routines and consistency.

When parents match their behaviors to what works best for a child, it is what developmental scientists call "goodness of fit." For example, parents who are naturally anxious may have to work hard not to be overly intrusive and protective on the playground with an active and exploratory child. However, a cautious child may need a bit more encouragement to explore, and they do not need us to make them more anxious by showing our fear and worry when they climb on a jungle gym.

Children often actively work to be different from their parents or other family members. This need for differentiating from the family and siblings is normal, although sometimes it can be unsettling. Often parents see this as rebelling, but it is usually temporary, and most parents and young adults share many of the same core values and become more similar as they mature. As we get to know our children's personalities, temperaments, strengths, and weaknesses, we may need to adjust our expectations. Our job is to help them find their way, not our way.

Have a Traveling Companion

Many people say it takes a village to raise a child, and we agree. It is certainly easier if parents have help, and sometimes parents have to actively reach out and ask for support. Social support is one of the best predictors of adult mental health, which is even more true in times of stress. Parents can get support from other parents, in moms' or dads' groups, through faith-based groups, or from other social outlets. Having responsible babysitters is important when children are young or single parents want to have a night out with friends. This allows parents time away from children, and it can be important for couples to have time just with each other. Paying for a sitter can be expensive, so trading off with other parents is a great idea, and children usually love spending time with other kids and getting some time away, too.

In our society today, it can be argued that we have lost our sense of community and connection. Most adults do not live near their parents, and many feel lonely and isolated. As we discussed previously, we are wired to connect. Being lonely is a risk factor for many forms of disease, such as high blood pressure, obesity, heart disease, depression, anxiety, and cognitive decline. Many families move close to their parents when their children are young because they realize the benefits of having a grandparent who lives close by. Building a sense of community is good for both parents and children. It gives parents the support they need, and children learn that they have connections and resources outside the home that they can turn to for advice and support or just fun.

It is also helpful to have a friend who has navigated a parenting stage before your children reach that age. They likely will have much wisdom to share, and often they will tell you about the mistakes they made, which can be critical information. Take advantage of weekend birthday parties and playground gatherings when kids are little and soccer games and school booster clubs as kids get older. These are great ways to meet other parents, who can be a lifeline when you are struggling with a particular issue.

Be a Safe Driver

Throughout this book, we have emphasized the need for parents to care for themselves to be good parents. It is difficult for parents to care for their children when their own needs are not met. It is not selfish for parents to take time for themselves to exercise, be in nature, or go on a weekend trip, as long as children are adequately cared for in their absence. In fact, children can learn that parents need breaks too, and they learn to be more independent when they have time away from moms and dads.

When children are young, it is hard to find time to exercise and get away for the weekend or take a break with a friend. This can be particularly challenging for working parents balancing careers and families. When children start going to school, parents have more time and can take advantage of this newfound freedom by building in time for themselves. Studies show that when adults take time for themselves to do something they enjoy each week, they feel like they have more time. Take control of your schedule when you're feeling overwhelmed and burned out. Make time for mindfulness, physical activity, and being in nature, all of which have calming effects on the brain. And note that most parents report some of their most enjoyable activities are being with other adults, not caring for their children. Parenting is hard work, stressful, and often not enjoy-able. Parents need to make time for activities outside the home to stay happy and healthy. We realize this is often a challenge, but be creative and find other families to help.

Like their children, parents need adequate sleep and regular physical activity to be healthy. Adults need at least 7 hours of sleep each night, and many need 8 or 9 hours to feel completely rested. They need about 150 minutes a week of moderate physical activity (30 minutes a day for 5 days). As we get older, strength training becomes more important, and we need muscle-strengthening activi-ties at least 2 days a week. There are many types of exercise, but the best kind is the one you will do! It can be as simple as a morning walk with a neighbor, an evening run with your dog, or an online yoga class twice a week. An excellent goal is to get outside weekly, with or without the kids. Family bike rides or trips to the park can be a great way to spend a Sunday afternoon.

Be Prepared for the Journey

Amanda remembers when she went out to dinner with her in-laws when her children were about 3 and 5. The grandparents let her and Mike finish dinner and have some time alone while they took the kids to the river park by the restaurant. When Mike and Amanda emerged from the restaurant and met up with them, both Caleb and Mollie were soaking wet! They had played in the fountains, having a ball in the hot Tulsa weather. That was one time Amanda did not hide her feelings as she realized they had no towels or dry clothes for her dripping children. But she did learn that she should always carry towels in the car, which has come in handy many times—after allowing her children to have spontaneous fun in a fountain or after a rainy soccer game. Having water bottles and snacks in the car or backpack can also be a lifesaver when caught in traffic or when unscheduled appointments keep us away from home longer than expected. Amanda and her kids have a propensity for motion sickness, so throw-up bags are always in their cars. When children are little, having diapers in the car can be a lifesaver, too, as can having small toys and games for unexpected waiting times. Parents need to be ready to use their imagination and start a game of I Spy, Telephone, or 20 Questions or simply tell a good story. Jennifer began keeping finger puppets in her bag after having to entertain 2-year-old Amy for an hour during an unplanned (by definition) trip to a busy emergency room for stitches one holiday weekend. We can't be prepared for everything, but it helps to be prepared for the most common situations.

Amanda's COVID story at the beginning of this chapter gave us one example of the demands on parents who are part of the sandwich generation, trying to meet the needs of their children and their aging parents at the same time. This is another situation in which it helps to prepare in advance, having conversations and making plans about how to handle the struggles many aging parents will face. Many financial and emotional crises can be avoided with careful and timely planning. It can be challenging to talk with parents and grandparents about difficult decisions, such as moving into assisted living or nursing care, but having these conversations before the situations become critical can relieve a lot of stress. The principles of crucial conversations discussed in Chapter 7 are useful in these situations. It is particularly helpful when the whole family can help out, including siblings who can share the burdens when parents age and have health problems.

PREPARING FOR THE UNEXPECTED

When Jennifer was 12 and her brother, Jeff, was 9, their mother was diagnosed with a rare and terminal cancer. Given only 3 to 5 months to live, she carried on through radiation and multiple surgeries as though the experts were wrong. And they were—to a point. For the next 2 years, Jennifer and Jeff continued going to school, enjoying time with their friends, playing the piano or guitar, and pretending nothing had changed. But the cancer finally won, and Jennifer's mother died 2 days after her 42nd birthday. Jennifer was 14, and Jeff was 11. Two weeks later, their father introduced them to the woman he would marry 4 months later and her children. Suddenly, everything changed: a new house, a new neighborhood, and a new school. One afternoon, Jennifer's father and stepmother also told her that her mother had gone to hell when she died, and she and Jeff were also headed to hell because they went to the wrong church. Jennifer walked into the bathroom, locked the door, looked at herself in the mirror, and thought, "They're wrong. I'm on my own now."

The next 4 years were not good. Looking back, Jennifer understood the basis for fairy tales like Cinderella and Hansel and Gretel. She remembers eating bologna or peanut butter sandwiches at home every night with her brother and stepsiblings while her father and stepmother went out to eat. There were no more piano lessons. When she was 16, they moved to another city, and she said goodbye to all her friends. Now she felt truly alone and betrayed by the father whose love she had always taken for granted. The one bright spot was school. She continued to do well in her classes in spite of working two to three jobs to pay for all her clothes, school supplies, food, and a car. She played the piano for the school choir and made a few new friends. When she was a few months short of graduation, her father and stepmother told her to pack up all her things and leave the house. She moved in with her boyfriend's older brother and his wife, whose children she often babysat, and gave the school her new address. She didn't know what she would do next or how she would pay for college.

Meanwhile, in another state, one of her mother's best friends began having dreams about Jennifer. After several sleepless nights, she called Jennifer's aunt, who called all the high schools Jennifer could be attending. The next thing she knew, the school counselor called her into her office and told Jennifer to call her aunt "collect" (this was before cell phones and free long-distance). Jennifer called, told her aunt and uncle what had happened, and they sent Jennifer a plane ticket to visit them the following weekend. They invited her to come and live with them after she graduated. They helped her find a job and made her feel at home. One day that summer, while driving under the overpass of a freeway, she had the strangest sensation of peace and calm. It was as if she had a glimpse of the future, a future when she would be happy and even grateful for the hardship and loss. She thought to herself that surely there were lessons embedded in these experiences that would make her stronger, wiser, and better. At that moment, everything changed. She wasn't afraid.

Jennifer knew she would survive and thrive because she had a solid foundation during the first part of her life. While far from perfect, during her first 12 years, her parents had given her unconditional love and the opportunity to have other supportive relationships. They had devoted time and resources to helping her develop her talents and skills during her early years. Even during the later difficult times, she had the support of many friends and her mother's friends. As in the fairy tales, she had a number of fairy godmothers whose help she gratefully accepted and whose love and support proved invaluable. The lessons of adversity and resilience were clearly outlined for Jennifer in her life and her family's history before she began to study the science of adversity and resilience. To quote our friend and colleague Michael Ungar, "No one is resilient alone."

As parents, we can try to prepare for the unexpected, but it is unexpected for a reason. Bad things happen even to good people. Adversity is real. When we deal with our ACEs or the ACEs of our children, we have no real choice but to keep moving forward, keep believing that things will be okay, and get the support we need to keep on going and to keep moving. It is never too late to make a change, admit we made a mistake, or mend a relationship. It takes time and hard work, but our children are worth it! We have learned that along the way, we will experience bumps, wrong turns, and accidents, and we will get lost. This is part of life and part of parenting. All we can do is learn from our mistakes, plan for what is next, and keep believing things will be okay.

ROAD MAP TO RESILIENCE AND KEY TAKEAWAYS

You may recall that earlier in the book, we invited you to choose the values you think are most important for children to develop (see the Activity section in Chapter 1). Now, we invite you to think back on that list and the resilient outcomes we have focused on throughout this book. In these final takeaways, we weave it all together, pointing out that resilient outcomes for our children can also be resilient outcomes for ourselves, giving us strength and courage during times of adversity on our parenting journey.

The first resilient outcome is *trust*. This is the foundation of the parent–child relationship and begins before children are even born. Parents have to conquer their fears and deal with past adversities so that they can enter into trusting relationships and be a source of trust for their children. This is manifested as unconditional love in the parent–child relationship and is the first and most important PACE. As our children grow, we need to trust not only ourselves but also that our children will be okay. We need to trust them and believe in them. This does not mean we are not aware of their mistakes and challenges, but we talk things through with them and are there for our kids, no matter what.

The next outcome is *courage*. When we are courageous as a parent, we tap into our source of inner strength and resolve. We persevere and keep going, no matter what. Advice Jennifer once received and found to be true is that "children follow strength." We need to be strong even when our children are struggling. Sometimes this means not revealing all the stress and worry we are feeling in the moment, staying calm, and assuring our children that they are safe with us along the way. As parents, we must encourage our children instead of discouraging them so that they will be able to journey out on their own someday and come and go and explore this world with a sense of confidence.

Third is *character*. Character is what we are building in our children so that they can be counted on to do the right thing—not because of external rewards or threats but because they have developed the values and principles to guide them in doing the right thing even when it is difficult. Developmental scientists call this *internalization*. We build character in ourselves when we push through difficult times and learn from our parenting successes and challenges. Recall that moral development progresses through stages (see Chapter 6) and that parents can help their children develop character by modeling it, labeling it, and regularly talking about it with them. This can be difficult for parents because it takes effort and intentionality. It is easier to say "because I said so" rather than always giving reasons and explanations for rules and consequences. But having conversations about right and wrong and why we value some behaviors over others builds character in ourselves and our children.

Fourth is *competence*. When our children develop skills and learn new things, they are becoming competent individuals, and they do not need us to do things for them that they can do for themselves. In fact, they will eventually become better at many things than we are. In this book, we encourage parents to build competence in themselves and their children through PACEs. In particular, we discuss the importance of having hobbies, being part of a group, engaging in lifelong learning, and providing quality educational opportunities. These PACEs encourage competence in various domains and can help children learn their strengths and how to collaborate with others in a group. As parents, we can expand on our parenting competence. You are doing this by reading this book! As we have discussed, parenting is a difficult job, one of the hardest. But there are many things we can do to become better parents, including taking parenting classes, reading books, and talking with other parents who have successfully navigated the parenting journey. We recommend all these strategies and finding what works best for you.

Fifth is *confidence*. If you are trustworthy, courageous, and competent, you should be confident as a parent. Believing you are competent and effective as a parent, what developmental scientists call *parenting efficacy*, helps you be a better parent. Being confident can be challenging during difficult times. Asking for help is never a sign of weakness, and it takes strength and confidence to admit when we need help or our children do. We cannot emphasize enough how helpful it can be to get expert advice from professionals when needed. Sometimes it takes hearing advice from someone else before children make a change or see things differently. It is important to remember that you are always the parent, and even when it is difficult, we have to remain the older adult in the relationship and provide support and stay calm when our children need us most. And keep believing in yourself.

The final resilient outcome is *purpose*. Our purpose as parents is to help our children navigate this world so that they also become trusting, courageous, competent, and confident adults with character. We do this by keeping them safe while letting them explore, having rules and limits, encouraging their independence while staying connected, and always communicating our unconditional love. As our children grow into adolescents and young adults, we want to help them set goals and have a sense of purpose in their lives. We want them to develop their identity separate from ours. We do this through conversations, support, and believing in them. As parents, we need to trust that our life has meaning, even when our kids leave home. And we want our children to know that they matter to us, no matter what, that we love them, and even when they leave home, we will always be their parents.

Congratulations! You've made it to the end of our parenting travel guide. No matter where you are on the journey, we hope you now feel more prepared and more confident. While it is impossible to be prepared for all the unexpected twists and turns, roadblocks, and detours along the way, you will be able to stay on track by focusing on the principles we've outlined. Indeed, some of the obstacles and hazards along the way can feel overwhelming. But parents have been raising children in difficult situations for as long as there have been humans. We hope that by sharing what we have learned about raising resilient children, you will agree that it is never too late to become resilient. Happy trails!

RESOURCES

Carter, C. (2011). *Raising happiness: 10 simple steps for more joyful kids and happier parents*. Ballantine Books.

Gottman, J. (2002). *The relationship cure: A 5-step guide to strengthening your marriage, family, and friendships*. Harmony.

Kabat-Zinn, J. (2016). *Mindfulness for beginners*. Sounds True.

ACEs and PACEs website: https://www.acesandpaces.com

REFERENCES

Ainsworth, M. D. S., Blehar, M. C., Waters, E., & Wall, S. (1978). *Patterns of attachment: A psychological study of the strange situation.* Erlbaum.

Anda, R. F., Felitti, V. J., Bremner, J. D., Walker, J. D., Whitfield, C., Perry, B. D., Dube, S. R., & Giles, W. H. (2006). The enduring effects of abuse and related adverse experiences in childhood. A convergence of evidence from neurobiology and epidemiology. *European Archives of Psychiatry and Clinical Neuroscience, 256*(3), 174–186. https://doi.org/10.1007/s00406-005-0624-4

Anderson, K. N., Swedo, E. A., Trinh, E., Ray, C. M., Krause, K. H., Verlenden, J. V., Clayton, H. B., Villaveces, A., Massetti, G. M., & Holditch Niolon, P. (2022). Adverse childhood experiences during the COVID-19 pandemic and associations with poor mental health and suicidal behaviors among high school students—Adolescent Behaviors and Experiences Survey, United States, January–June 2021. *Morbidity and Mortality Weekly Report, 71*(41), 1301–1305. https://doi.org/10.15585/mmwr.mm7141a2

Aupperle, R. L., Morris, A. S., Silk, J. S., Criss, M. M., Judah, M. R., Eagleton, S. G., Kirlic, N., Byrd-Craven, J., Phillips, R., & Alvarez, R. P. (2016). Neural responses to maternal praise and criticism: Relationship to depression and anxiety symptoms in high-risk adolescent girls. *NeuroImage: Clinical, 11*, 548–554. https://doi.org/10.1016/j.nicl.2016.03.009

Baglivio, M. T., Epps, N., Swartz, K., Huq, M. S., Sheer, A., & Hardt, N. S. (2014). The prevalence of adverse childhood experiences (ACE) in the lives of juvenile offenders. *Journal of Juvenile Justice*, 3(2). https://www.prisonpolicy.org/scans/Prevalence_of_ACE.pdf

Baumrind, D. (1971). Current patterns of parental authority. *Developmental Psychology*, 4(1, Pt. 2), 1–103. https://doi.org/10.1037/h0030372

Bellis, M. A., Hughes, K., Ford, K., Ramos Rodriguez, G., Sethi, D., & Passmore, J. (2019, September 3). Life course health consequences and associated annual costs of adverse childhood experiences across Europe and North America: A systematic review and meta-analysis. *The Lancet*, 4(10), e517–e528. https://doi.org/10.1016/S2468-2667(19)30145-8

Berk, L. (2015). *Child development*. Pearson.

Bitsko, R. H., Claussen, A. H., Lichstein, J., Black, L. I., Jones, S. E., Danielson, M. L., Hoenig, J. M., Davis Jack, S. P., Brody, D. J., Gyawali, S., Maenner, M. J., Warner, M., Holland, K. M., Perou, R., Crosby, A. E., Blumberg, S. J., Avenevoli, S., Kaminski, J. W., & Ghandour, R. M. (2022). Mental health surveillance among children—United States, 2013–2019. *MMWR Supplements*, 71(2), 1–42. https://doi.org/10.15585/mmwr.su7102a1

Bowlby, J. (2008). *A secure base: Parent–child attachment and healthy human development*. Basic Books.

Brazelton, T. B., & Sparrow, J. D. (2005). *Understanding sibling rivalry—The Brazelton way*. Da Capo Lifelong Books.

Brummelman, E., Nelemans, S. A., Thomaes, S., & Orobio de Castro, B. (2017). When parents' praise inflates, children's self-esteem deflates. *Child Development*, 88(6), 1799–1809. https://doi.org/10.1111/cdev.12936

Centers for Disease Control and Prevention. (2023). *Anxiety and depression in children*. https://www.cdc.gov/childrensmentalhealth/depression.html

Davidson, R. J., Kabat-Zinn, J., Schumacher, J., Rosenkranz, M., Muller, D., Santorelli, S. F., Urbanowski, F., Harrington, A., Bonus, K., & Sheridan, J. F. (2003). Alterations in brain and immune function produced by mindfulness meditation. *Psychosomatic Medicine*, 65(4), 564–570. https://doi.org/10.1097/01.PSY.0000077505.67574.E3

Davis, J. L. (2008). *Treating post-trauma nightmares: A cognitive behavioral approach*. Springer.

Dayton, J., & Faris, V. (Directors). (2006). *Little miss sunshine* [Film]. Searchlight Pictures.

de Moor, G. (2011). Supporting moral development: The Virtues Project™. *Reclaiming Children and Youth*, 20(2), 54–58.

Duncan, L. G., Coatsworth, J. D., & Greenberg, M. T. (2009). A model of mindful parenting: Implications for parent-child relationships and prevention research. *Clinical Child and Family Psychology Review*, *12*(3), 255–270. https://doi.org/10.1007/s10567-009-0046-3

Dweck, C. S. (2017). The journey to children's mindsets—and beyond. *Child Development Perspectives*, *11*(2), 139–144. https://doi.org/10.1111/cdep.12225

Eckert-Lind, C., Busch, A. S., Petersen, J. H., Biro, F. M., Butler, G., Bräuner, E. V., & Juul, A. (2020). Worldwide secular trends in age at pubertal onset assessed by breast development among girls: A systematic review and meta-analysis. *JAMA Pediatrics*, *174*(4), e195881. https://doi.org/10.1001/jamapediatrics.2019.5881

Erikson, E. H. (1993). *Childhood and society*. Norton.

Felitti, V. J., Anda, R. F., Nordenberg, D., Williamson, D. F., Spitz, A. M., Edwards, V., Koss, M. P., & Marks, J. S. (1998). Relationship of childhood abuse and household dysfunction to many of the leading causes of death in adults: The Adverse Childhood Experiences (ACE) Study. *American Journal of Preventive Medicine*, *14*(4), 245–258. https://doi.org/10.1016/S0749-3797(98)00017-8

Fraiberg, S., Adelson, E., & Shapiro, V. (2018). Ghosts in the nursery: A psychoanalytic approach to the problems of impaired infant–mother relationships. In J. Raphael-Leff (Ed.), *Parent–infant psychodynamics: Wild things, mirrors and ghosts* (pp. 87–117). Routledge. https://doi.org/10.4324/9780429478154-10

Gardner, H. (2006). *Multiple intelligences: New horizons in theory and practice*. Basic Books.

Gershoff, E. T. (2013). Spanking and child development: We know enough now to stop hitting our children. *Child Development Perspectives*, *7*(3), 133–137. https://doi.org/10.1111/cdep.12038

Gershoff, E. T., Goodman, G. S., Miller-Perrin, C. L., Holden, G. W., Jackson, Y., & Kazdin, A. E. (2018). The strength of the causal evidence against physical punishment of children and its implications for parents, psychologists, and policymakers. *American Psychologist*, *73*(5), 626–638. https://doi.org/10.1037/amp0000327

Gottman, J. (2011). *Raising an emotionally intelligent child*. Simon & Schuster.

Harter, S. (2015). *The construction of the self* (2nd ed.). Guilford Press.

Hayward, C., Killen, J. D., Wilson, D. M., Hammer, L. D., Litt, I. F., Kraemer, H. C., Haydel, F., Varady, A., & Taylor, C. B. (1997). Psychiatric risk associated with early puberty in adolescent girls. *Journal of the American Academy of Child & Adolescent Psychiatry*, *36*(2), 255–262.

Hoffman, K. T., Marvin, R. S., Cooper, G., & Powell, B. (2006). Changing toddlers' and preschoolers' attachment classifications: The Circle of Security intervention. *Journal of Consulting and Clinical Psychology*, 74(6), 1017–1026. https://doi.org/10.1037/0022-006X.74.6.1017

Hughes, D. L., Fisher, C., & Cabrera, N. J. (2020). Talking to children about racism: Breaking the cycle of bias and violence starts at home. *Child & Family Blog*. https://www.childandfamilyblog.com/child-development/talking-to-children-about-racism

Kabat-Zinn, J. (2005). *Wherever you go, there you are: Mindfulness meditation in everyday life* (10th ed.). Hachette Books.

Kohlberg, L. (1985). *The psychology of moral development: Essays on moral development*. Harper & Row.

Kondo, M. (2014). *The life-changing magic of tidying up: The Japanese art of decluttering and organizing*. Ten Speed Press.

Lieberman, A. F., Padrón, E., Van Horn, P., & Harris, W. W. (2005). Angels in the nursery: The intergenerational transmission of benevolent parental influences. *Infant Mental Health Journal*, 26(6), 504–520. https://doi.org/10.1002/imhj.20071

Ludington-Hoe, S. M., & Swinth, J. Y. (1996). Developmental aspects of kangaroo care. *Journal of Obstetric, Gynecologic, and Neonatal Nursing*, 25(8), 691–703. https://doi.org/10.1111/j.1552-6909.1996.tb01483.x

Marcia, J. E. (1966). Development and validation of ego-identity status. *Journal of Personality and Social Psychology*, 3(5), 551–558. https://doi.org/10.1037/h0023281

Marvin, R., Cooper, G., Hoffman, K., & Powell, B. (2002). The Circle of Security project: Attachment-based intervention with caregiver-pre-school child dyads. *Attachment & Human Development*, 4(1), 107–124. https://doi.org/10.1080/14616730252982491

Masten, A. S. (2015). *Ordinary magic: Resilience in development*. Guilford Press.

McKelvey, L. M., Whiteside-Mansell, L., Conners-Burrow, N. A., Swindle, T., & Fitzgerald, S. (2016). Assessing adverse experiences from infancy through early childhood in home visiting programs. *Child Abuse & Neglect*, 51, 295–302. https://doi.org/10.1016/j.chiabu.2015.09.008

Morris, A. S., Hays-Grudo, J., Zapata, M. I., Treat, A., & Kerr, K. L. (2021). Adverse and protective childhood experiences and parenting attitudes: The role of cumulative protection in understanding resilience. *Adversity and Resilience Science, 2*(3), 181–192. https://doi.org/10.1007/s42844-021-00036-8

Osmanoglu, D. E. (2019). Child abuse and children's strategies to cope with abuse. *World Journal of Education, 9*(1), 28–37. https://dx.doi.org/10.5430/wje.v9n1p28

Paruthi, S., Brooks, L. J., D'Ambrosio, C., Hall, W. A., Kotagal, S., Lloyd, R. M., Malow, B. A., Maski, K., Nichols, C., Quan, S. F., Rosen, C. L., Troester, M. M., & Wise, M. S. (2016). Consensus statement of the American Academy of Sleep Medicine on the recommended amount of sleep for healthy children: Methodology and discussion. *Journal of Clinical Sleep Medicine, 12*(1), 1549–1561. https://doi.org/10.5664/jcsm.6288

Patterson, K., Grenny, J., McMillan, R., & Switzler, A. (2012). *Crucial conversations: Tools for talking when stakes are high* (2nd ed.). McGraw-Hill.

Pennebaker, J. W. (2018). Expressive writing in psychological science. *Perspectives on Psychological Science, 13*(2), 226–229. https://doi.org/10.1177/1745691617707315

Popkin, M. H. (2014). *Active parenting: A parent's guide to raising happy and successful children* (4th ed.). Active Parenting Press.

Popkin, M. H., Morris, A. S., Slocum, R., & Hubbs-Tait, L. (2017). *Active parenting first five years: Parent's guide*. Active Parenting Press.

Popov, L. K., Popov, D., & Kavelin, J. (1997). *The family virtues guide: Simple ways to bring out the best in our children and ourselves*. Plume.

Ratliff, E. L., Kerr, K. L., Misaki, M., Cosgrove, K. T., Moore, A. J., DeVille, D. C., Silk, J. S., Barch, D. M., Tapert, S. F., Simmons, W. K., Bodurka, J., & Morris, A. S. (2021). Into the unknown: Examining neural representations of parent–adolescent interactions. *Child Development, 92*(6), e1361–e1376. https://doi.org/10.1111/cdev.13635

Snyder, J., Low, S., Bullard, L., Schrepferman, L., Wachlarowicz, M., Marvin, C., & Reed, A. (2013). Effective parenting practices: Social interaction learning theory and the role of emotion coaching and mindfulness. In R. E. Larzelere, A. S. Morris, & A. W. Harrist (Eds.), *Authoritative parenting: Synthesizing nurturance and discipline for optimal child development* (pp. 189–210). American Psychological Association. https://doi.org/10.1037/13948-009

Spock, B. (1957). *Baby and child care* (2nd ed.). Pocket Books.

Tamis-LeMonda, C. S., Way, N., Hughes, D., Yoshikawa, H., Kalman, R. K., & Niwa, E. Y. (2008). Parents' goals for children: The dynamic coexistence of individualism and collectivism in cultures and individuals. *Social Development*, *17*(1), 183–209. https://dx.doi.org/10.1111/j.1467-9507.2007.00419.x

Teens and Pornography. (2023, January 10). *Common Sense*. https://www.commonsensemedia.org/research/teens-and-pornography

van Der Kolk, B. (2014). *The body keeps the score: Brain, mind, and body in the healing of trauma*. Penguin.

Vygotsky, L. S. (1978). *Mind in society: The development of higher psychological processes*. Harvard University Press.

Wade, M., Zeanah, C. H., Fox, N. A., & Nelson, C. A. (2020). Social communication deficits following early-life deprivation and relation to psychopathology: A randomized clinical trial of foster care. *Journal of Child Psychology and Psychiatry, and Allied Disciplines*, *61*(12), 1360–1369. https://doi.org/10.1111/jcpp.13222

Wade, R., Jr., Shea, J. A., Rubin, D., & Wood, J. (2014). Adverse childhood experiences of low-income urban youth. *Pediatrics*, *134*(1), e13–e20. https://doi.org/10.1542/peds.2013-2475

Yamaoka, Y., & Bard, D. E. (2019). Positive parenting matters in the face of early adversity. *American Journal of Preventive Medicine*, *56*(4), 530–539. https://doi.org/10.1016/j.amepre.2018.11.018

Zeanah, C. H., Fox, N. A., & Nelson, C. A. (2019). Recovery from severe deprivation: The Bucharest early intervention project. *Journal of the American Academy of Child Psychiatry*, *58*(10), S300–S301.

INDEX

Alcohol use and abuse
athletic goals and, 53
consequences for, 197
discussing, 227–228
in early adulthood, 210, 227–228
by parent, 145–146, 227
resources on preventing, 239
setting boundaries on, 224–225
Allowance, 157–158
Alternatives, thinking through, 214
Altruism, 49
American Academy of Pediatrics, 83, 85
American Psychological Association, 59
Amygdala, 213
Anda, Robert, 32–33
"Angels" in the nursery, 80, 93, 249
Anger, 81–82, 90, 114, 124, 130
Anterior insula, 213
Anxiety, 19, 177–178, 202, 233
Anxious attachment, 76
Anxious parenting, 16
Apologizing, 124, 220
Approval, love vs., 246–247
Argumentative responses, 222
Attachment
in adolescence, 194
and exploration, 76–78
and faith, 245
separation versus, 17, 71, 74–76
and unconditional love, 246
Attachment parenting, 75
Attachment problems, 18
Attention, 124
Attention-deficit/hyperactivity disorder
(ADHD), 134, 135
Attractiveness, 41
Audiobooks, 158
Auditory processing disorders, 135
Authoritarian parenting style, 13
Authoritative parenting style, 13,
139–140
Authority, of stepparents, 186–187
Automatic responses, 113
Automobile safety for teen drivers, 239

Autonomy
balancing boundaries and, 17, 180
in early adolescence, 173, 179, 183
in late adolescence and early
adulthood, 218
need for protection and, 14
Avoidant attachment, 75–76
Awareness of emotions, 124

Babies. *See* Infancy
Baby blues, 71
"Bad touch" conversations, 127–128
Balanced parenting approach
breaking cycle of adversity with, 54
to build child's resilience, 3–4, 12–15
to build parent's resilience, 242–248
case vignettes, 7–8, 23–24
defined, 12
by developmental stage, 15–17
in early adolescence, 21–22, 178–184
in early childhood, 19–20, 105–111
in infancy, 18–19, 70–76
in late adolescence and young
adulthood, 22–23, 214, 216–222
in middle childhood, 20–21,
136–144
outcomes of, 17–23
principles of, 16
resources on, 27
Setting Your Destination activity,
24–27
in toddlerhood, 19, 70–71, 76–79
for unexpected situations, 87–90
Bar mitzvahs and bat mitzvahs, 22
Baumrind, Diana, 12–13, 139
Beauty standards, 162–163
Bedtime routines, 50, 83, 126, 173,
181–182
Behavioral indicators, of crucial
conversations, 220
Behavioral needs of children, 12
Behavioral problems, 38
Behavior of child, impact of parenting
style on, 12–13
Being with child, 193–195

Belonging, 171–172

Benevolence, 43, 48–49

Best friends, 47–48, 105, 142–143

Bias, 5–6

"Big sex talk," 151, 189, 227

Birthday parties, 121

Blame, 144, 160, 161, 198, 251

Blended families, 186–188

Bodily-kinesthetic intelligence, 149–150

Body image problems, 162–163

The Body Keeps the Score (van Der Kolk), 113

"Bonus book" concept, 101–103

Boot camp model, 126

Boundaries, 49

  balancing autonomy and, 17, 180

  in blended families, 187

  conversations about, 183–184

  in early adolescence, 176, 179

  for teens, 224–225

Bowlby, John, 75

Boys

  physical development of, 212

  puberty for, 135, 161, 173

Brain development

  in early adolescence, 174, 176, 188

  effects of ACEs on, 37–38

  impact of experience on, 39–40

  in infancy, 65–66

  in late adolescence, 212–214

  parental influence on child's, 212–213

Bray, James, 187

Brazelton, T. Berry, 155

Breastfeeding, 63, 65, 98

Brothers Grimm, 11

Budgeting, 231

Bullying, 34, 148–149, 153, 155, 165, 233

Bystanders, 148–149

Caffeine, 173

Calderón, Rey, 61–62, 79

Calmness, 113, 120, 124, 130, 243–245

Camps, 150–151

Career-boosting hobbies, 53–54

Caregivers

  conflicts between, 24–25

  finding alternate, 115. *See also* Child care providers

Caring, rule-setting as, 196–197

Carpooling, 196

Categorization, 118

Cause-and-effect connections, 103–104, 174

Center for Gender Diversity, 192

Centers for Disease Control and Prevention, 63, 191

ChAACEs. *See* Childhood adaptations to ACEs

Character, 17, 19–20, 108–110, 121, 262–263

Charitable donations, 231

Check-in conversations, 22

  in early adolescence, 147, 149, 165–166, 197

  in late adolescence/early adulthood, 213, 217, 226–228

Child and family services agency, 81

Child care, balancing self-care and, 13, 111, 143–144, 164

Child care providers. *See also* Grandparents

  choosing, for infants and toddlers, 93, 99

  in community, 255–256

  taking turns as, 143–144

  toilet training practices of, 68–69

Childhood adaptations to ACEs (ChAACEs)

  activities on, 166–168, 203–205

  breaking cycle of adversity by identifying, 145–146, 250–251

  in early adolescence, 198–199, 203–205

  GrAACEs and, 184, 185

  of parents, 145–146, 166–168, 184, 185

ABOUT THE AUTHORS

Amanda Sheffield Morris, PhD, is a regents professor and the George Kaiser Family Foundation Chair in the Department of Psychology at Oklahoma State University. She was a coinvestigator on the multisite National Institutes of Health (NIH)–funded Adolescent Brain Cognitive Development study and is a principal investigator on a similar study of infant and child development, the Healthy Brain and Child Development study. Dr. Morris has authored numerous articles and chapters on child and adolescent development and the neuroscience of emotion regulation and parenting. She is coeditor of two books, *Authoritative Parenting: Synthesizing Nurturance and Discipline for Optimal Child Development* and *The Cambridge Handbook of Parenting: Interdisciplinary Research and Application*. With Jennifer Hays-Grudo, she is coauthor of *Adverse and Protective Childhood Experiences: A Developmental Perspective*.

Jennifer Hays-Grudo, PhD, is a regents professor of psychiatry and behavioral sciences at the Center for Health Sciences at Oklahoma State University, where she directs the Center for Integrative Research on Childhood Adversity, a National Institutes of Health–funded center addressing the effects of early life experience on health and development. She cochaired the Oklahoma Legislative Task Force on Trauma-Informed Care. Dr. Hays-Grudo has published numerous scientific articles on the effects of adversity on children and families, risk-taking in adolescents, and the effects of nutrition and hormone therapy on quality of life and cognition in postmenopausal women. She is coauthor with Amanda Sheffield Morris of *Adverse and Protective Childhood Experiences: A Developmental Perspective*, and is the founding editor-in-chief of the journal *Adversity and Resilience Science*.